I Won't Be Shaken

A Story of
Overcoming
the Odds

Joshua Loyd Fox

Published by Watertower Hill Publishing, LLC
5 Charter St.
Exeter, NH 03833
www.watertowerhillpublishing.com

Copyright © 2020 by J.L. Fox
www.jlfoxbooks.com

Cover design by J.L. Fox.
Interior design by J.L. Fox.

ISBN: 978-1-7362983-0-5

Library of Congress Control Number: 2021918454

Permissions:

Stand in Your Love *words and music by Josh Baldwin and Bethel Music. Copyright ©, 2018. All reasonable efforts were made to contact the copyright holders before publishing date of this book.*

TedTalk quotes by Dr. Nadine Harris-Burke *Copyright © 2015. All reasonable efforts were made to contact the copyright holders before publishing date of this book.*

www.beautyafterbruises.org *Copyright © The Foundation for Enhancing Communities. TFEC.org. All reasonable efforts were made to contact any copyright holders before the publishing date of this book.*

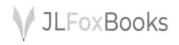

This book is dedicated to my best friend, Mary Elizabeth,
Who once kept me from walking into a wall while my nose was in a
book.

This book is also dedicated to my children.
You are the light of my world, and the reason I do
Everything.
You, all of you, are the best of me.

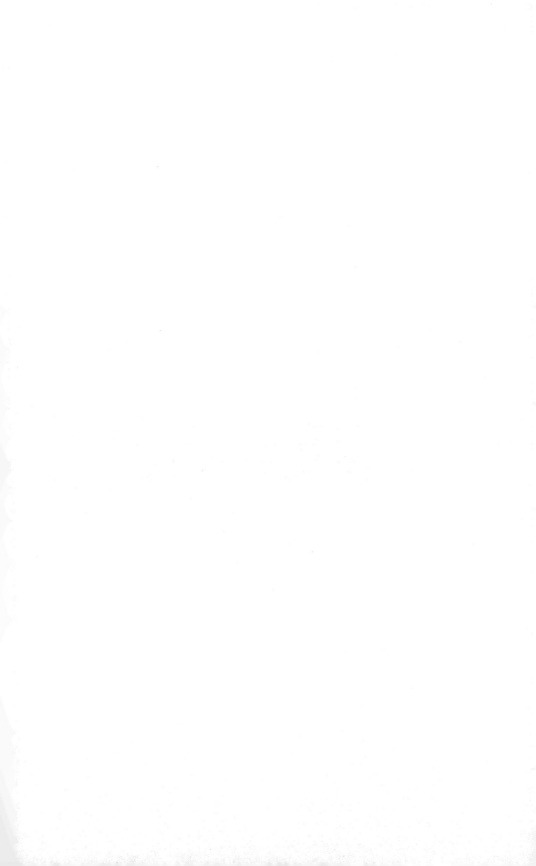

Yes, my soul, find rest in God;
my hope comes from him.
Truly he is my rock and my salvation;
he is my fortress, I will not be shaken.

--Psalms 62: 5-6 NIV

"When darkness tries to roll over my bones
When sorrow comes to steal the joy I own
When brokenness and pain is all I know
Oh, I won't be shaken, no I won't be shaken."
--Stand in Your Love
Song by Bethel Music
Sung by Josh Baldwin

First Introduction

I am, first and foremost, a storyteller. An orator of Tall Tales. A collector of life lessons if you will. My life has been consumed with stories, and I've used them primarily as an escape from my actual circumstances. All my life, I have wanted to do nothing but tell my stories to rapt audiences and share with them the joy these narratives bring me. Of all my stories, this one is the most important.

This particular tale begins the year I celebrated my fortieth birthday. It was a milestone that went by quickly; it was largely unnoticed by the world.

As I tell this tale, I have prematurely gray hair. I wear a full beard, which also shows signs of gray. I'm 6 feet, 3 inches tall, dark, and handsome. People who know me always remark on how intelligent I am. I'm not sure if it's because of anything other than my well-spoken nature and ability to carry on a conversation. However, I *do* have an eidetic memory. My eyes are dark brown, and my mother used to tell me that they looked as if they were made from wood grain.

I know all these things because that's what my eyes see when I look in the mirror, but there is no way these things could ever describe who and what I am. When I look around the coffee shop I'm sitting in, I don't think that logically, I'm different than any person here. Every person here has problems, everyone has relationships of some form, and everyone is loved by God. I went a long time in my life not believing most of that. I went through a large portion of this lifetime thinking I was different—and not in a good way. I feel no real connection with anyone here today, or anyone in the world, for that matter.

When you hate yourself, it's incredibly difficult to rise to who God made you to be and fulfill your purpose. My purpose is to write. I've always heard that when you aren't fulfilling your purpose, you don't have joy. And when you can't feel joy, you will never be happy. I'm finally learning how to be happy.

For the last two years, my life has been completely turned upside down. Each and every day has been a battle of defeats and conquests. My emotions have ridden that roller coaster for better or worse, to the point where I almost ended it all. I'm not afraid to admit it.

See, I gave God a final ultimatum: He had to bless my life in the way that I wanted Him to or else I would kill myself. It was my last act of defiance. My whole life had been a struggle, every single day, and I was tired. I was so tired of it all. I was weary in my bones and my mind could not fathom going any further. If God had blessed my life that day in a big way, I wouldn't have noticed. I had made up my mind— and if there is one thing I am, it's decisive—but I was to learn a very important lesson that day and every day following it. It was not yet in His time. I was on a razor's edge. I could not see the future He had in store for me. If I had, I would have been scared out of my mind.

I had no idea that by the time I told this story, God would give me the miracle that I had desired for what seemed like forever. As I sat down to tell this particular tale, I had no idea that my life would be bigger, grander, and much richer than I could ever have imagined. I just had to go through fire to get there— a fire that almost destroyed me completely.

This is my story.

Second Introduction

The whole week that started this process, this story, the reason I'm even telling it, happened in June of 2019.

I didn't sleep most of that week. I hardly ate. I spent every waking moment in such a severe depression, I don't know how I functioned. I would watch YouTube videos of everything from sermons of your dreams coming true, to learning about the Law of Attraction. I was manically writing notes down in notebooks about how to make my life better, and how to make it make sense, and how to change my destiny.

I made plans after plans, scribbled in spidery scrawl across my notebooks, of making my dreams come true. I only left the apartment, that whole week, for one thing.

Every afternoon, I would go on a walk. I would walk mile after mile. I would be drenched in sweat from the hot Florida weather. I would get rained on, and sunburnt. I didn't stop. I walked until I had half dollar sized blisters on the bottom of my feet. And the next day, I would walk again, making the blisters bleed. During the walks, I would rail at God. Cursing him because everyone around me was being blessed. Where were my blessings? Why was I all alone? Why did no one love me? Why the hell did I have to go through so much in my life, when millions of others had it so much better?

I cried and screamed at God in prayer about taking my parents when I was young. I cried and cursed him for my ruined relationships. And then I would apologize to Him and beg for a miracle in my life. I would put on my headphones and listen to my "Peace" playlist. Full of Christian music, but one song stuck out more than the others. Josh Baldwin's, "Stand In your Love". I listened to it over and over, trying to suck the meaning of the words into my soul. I even made it my ringtone on my phone for when anyone would call me or text me. I wanted that reminder at all times, that everything was going to be alright. But no one called. No one texted me that week.

The week before, I had lost my job, and was getting kicked out of my apartment.

But I made no plans for moving out of my apartment. Or to get a new job. I was applying, but nothing was happening. I screamed at God for that as well. Where the hell was He taking me? Hadn't I put it all in His hands? Where were His answers, and His signs? I listened to gospel music all week. I prayed and prayed. I walked and walked. I watched every sermon I could about how to make God hear me, and do something, damn it! I told Him I was trusting Him. I told Him that His will be done. And then I watched movies that would make me cry on purpose. I cried and cried that week. I thought it was cleansing me, but it just made it worse.

And then on Thursday, during my walk, and talking to God in a complete mental black hole, I had an epiphany.

I would make a deal with God.

As I walked around the beautiful neighborhood I lived in, amongst greenery and unimaginable tranquility that I didn't notice, I told God point blank that if He didn't make a miracle happen by Sunday night, I would kill myself.

It was my last act of defiance, and my last attempt to make it all better. As soon as I made the deal with God, I felt a calm and peace come over me like a bucket of ice-cold water. I instantly heard the birds chirping and saw the beauty of the green golf course my neighborhood surrounded. The tightness in my chest dissipated and my headache, which had been buzzing for days, went away. I could feel my eyes dilating, and my skin pinpricked with sweat from the hot sun. I smiled. I had my answer.

I walked one more four-mile lap and went back to my apartment with a spring in my step. I almost felt happy. I had a plan. A life of living by one plan or another had given me an anchor when things got rough. I learned to be disciplined years before. And now, I wasn't awash in uncertainty anymore. I got on the computer and found on the black web the best way to commit suicide. This time it wasn't going to be running headfirst into a wall in a jail cell in Utah.

No, this time it would be perfectly thought out and rigorously followed.

That night, even if God had granted me my desires and made some miracle happen, I didn't care. I was going to kill myself on Sunday night. I ate a big dinner that night and got on Amazon and ordered what I would need to get the job done. I had a delivery date the next day, and that, too, was perfect. This was all coming together nicely.

I will not write here the way in which I was going to do it, as I don't want to give the idea to any reader who may be thinking of doing the same thing. But it was fool-proof. I got back out my notebook and listed the plan in beautiful handwriting this time. I was calm, collected, and driven. The old spark came back. I would not fail in this.

Friday came, and I was happy. My plan was listed, and organized, and to be honest, that day, I didn't even think about it. I read my bible and watched some funny movies. I didn't even apply for jobs or plan to move out of the apartment. I could breathe. My worries would soon be over. I slept Friday night like a baby. I slept for over 12 hours. My mind, at least, was at peace.

And then, I woke up Saturday morning.

I had an overwhelming urge to talk to someone. I didn't know who, but a voice in my head was screaming at me to be heard. I felt like that voice had been there the whole time, but it wasn't until I was able to sleep deeply that I could hear it.

It was 7am on Saturday, June 29th. I took out my phone and looked through the contacts. And that's when I saw her name. My best friend since middle school. My sister-in-arms. The real love of my life.

Mary.

She had been in my life since I was 12 years old. Twenty-eight years I have known this woman. We had met out at Boys Ranch, the orphanage I grew up in, when I was in the 7th grade. She was a staff girl there, and while we weren't necessarily close at the Ranch, afterwards, we had shared everything with each other. She had been married to her husband for more than 20 years. She had 5 kids, and I loved her completely. She could never do any wrong in my eyes.

She knew everything that had happened to me in Florida. Hell, she knew when I had lost my virginity. More than anyone else in my life, she had been there the whole time, and I loved her completely. Writing this, I'm itching to reach for my phone just to call her. But I can't. I have to get out what happened next.

It was before 6am where she lived. I knew she loved to sleep in on the weekends. All her kids were at least teenagers, and she had gone through years of having no rest. At the present, she was a nurse with a very specific specialty. She had been featured in national magazines for helping women and men with pelvic floor weakness and muscle control loss in the pelvic region. She was tops in her field, and I loved the fact that after years of being a stay at home mom, doting on her children and her unappreciative husband, she had pulled herself up and was making something of herself. I didn't think she would answer the phone, but I called anyway. I had to quiet the screaming voice in my mind. So, I dialed.

She picked up on the first ring.

I just blurted out to her that I had made a plan, ordered the equipment to make it work, and that this was the last time I was going to talk to her. She didn't get upset at me. She didn't rail at me or tell me not to do it. She knew me better than that. She asked me one question. In her soft, quiet voice, she said,

"Have you told your brother"?

I started to cry so hard I couldn't stop shaking. I'm tearing up right now writing this. Hearing her beautiful voice in that phone, a thousand miles away from me, I realized I hadn't even thought about the people in my life who did love me. The people in my life who had been there for so many years I lost count. I didn't think about my brother. I didn't think about my children.

I was hell bent on ending the pain and the burden of my horrible life. I forgot all about the love I did have. Mary simply listened to me cry and made me promise to call Jasper before I did anything. She told me that she loved me, and that I wasn't the first Boys Rancher to call her with the same plan. I swear to this day that meeting Mary so many years before was because of this day.

God saw this day 28 years before and made me start to love a girl with a head full of curly hair and a sarcastic mouth, and a heart of pure gold.

I was in my living room, my body quaking in deep sobs when I hung up with her. I didn't want to die. I was never afraid of death before, and am not afraid to die now, but I did not want to die that day.

No one knew my story.

Not in its entirety. I thought no one cared if I lived or died, but I was so wrong. I had actually been surrounded by love my entire life. I was too caught up in my circumstances to see it. My God loved me and showed me that love by putting people in my life to love me despite how dense I was. How ego-centric and caught up in my own world to see it. This life was beautiful. Every bit of it. I was at the bottom of a deep, deep hole, but I would come out of it.

I still had lessons to learn, but within six weeks, everything would be turned around. I had to go through a little more hell after that day, but by September, I would be whole, and finally at peace. It was still a journey, and there was still a little bit more to go, but when I cried my last sob that morning, and hung up the phone with Mary, the clouds were parting, and the sunshine was breaking though.

I will love that woman for the rest of my life and will do absolutely anything for her. She saved my life. I realized she had saved it 28 years before by being my friend and loving me, she just didn't know it would take almost three decades for her job with me to be done.

28 years prior, I met her as a 7th grader, when she stopped me from walking into a wall between the middle school and high school wings of my school. I was reading a really good book, as I did most days back then, and I wasn't watching where I was going. She was new at the school, and pulling me out of the way of running head first into a concrete wall made her stand out in my mind. As did the next thing she said.

"You'll never have a girlfriend with your nose always in a book," she said. I laughed, and wondered who this girl was.

Whoever else comes into my life, in whatever capacity, for the rest of it, Mary will always be my best friend. How do you properly thank someone like that who saved your life with a phone call? I later asked her why she was awake so early that morning, and all she could tell me was that a voice woke her up, and she had her phone in her hand when I called. It was on silent mode, and didn't even buzz in her hand, but she saw my call immediately, and answered. When we discussed it, a year later, we were all baffled by it all.

But, it did not surprise her at all, at the time.

Nor did what came next.

Chapter 1

I was born in Berkeley, California in June of 1979. My father was 54 years old, and my mother, a college student at UC Berkeley, was 23. I have one biological brother, Jasper, who had been born in San Francisco 14 months prior to the hot summer day that I came crying into my dysfunctional life.

I really have no idea what was going on in my parent's lives in 1979. Circumstances would prove that no one really knew what was going on. My father was a Baptist preacher. I don't think he ran a church, but I did learn that he had a street ministry, on the corner right across from the entrance to the University of California, Berkeley. He taught the Word to the wayward youth of the late 1970's in one of the most liberal places on the planet. Apparently, this is how he met my biological mother, as well as her roommate, Linda.

My father was divorced from his first wife, Anne, who he had been married to for over thirty years. They had had four children, all of whom were grown and starting their own families and careers. From what I gather, all four of them were marginally successful, and lived lives better than what I grew up in. I only met some of my older siblings a couple of times when I was little, as they were not very happy with my father starting a new family. I can imagine there was quite a bit of animosity there, but of course, that wasn't my brother's or my fault. My father made those decisions. And we, in turn, had to suffer for them.

I learned much later in life, that when I was about six weeks old, my biological mother, Margrit, took Jasper and I to visit her parents in Boston. She had grown up there, with my grandparents, Norman, and Vera Wolff.

Norman had been an American soldier stationed in Germany after WW2. There, he had met my grandmother, who had already had my mother. My grandmother, Vera, went to her grave with the knowledge of who my biological grandfather was, and the only thing anyone knew was that he, too, had been a British soldier. There are family rumors that his name had been Wally or Walter, but there is no concrete information, and only one grainy picture of the man.

My adoptive grandfather, Norman Wolff, fell in love with my grandmother, and married her. I was later told that he also approached Wally, or whatever his name was, and told him in no uncertain terms that he planned on adopting my mother. I believe some fisticuffs may have been threatened. Knowing my grandfather, I wouldn't doubt if for a second.

So, he brought his new wife and newly adopted daughter back to the US, and they were naturalized here. I know there was a lot more to the story, but I don't know it all, and my mother's family doesn't talk about it much.

They called my mother "Mushi" which in German is the shortened version of 'Momma's girl'. I love that they all called her that, as I have never met my mother and grandmother together in real life, and I am in awe that they must have had an amazing relationship.

My mother eventually had two more sisters and a brother. My grandparents stayed together for the next 50 odd years. I met them twice in my late twenties. By then, most of the damage had been done, but it was interesting to learn that I had had so much history with this family, all the way across the country from what I grew up knowing. This family would become pivotal to my life much later.

When I was six weeks old and my mother brought my brother and I to visit, she made the decision to abandon me there with my grandparents, who didn't even have a diaper. I found out, again, much later in life, that my biological mother was removing me from the picture to work things out with my father.

He had assumed, from something that happened that only the two of them know about, that I wasn't his biological child. He even told his own family that fact. So, my mother dropped me off with her parents for six months and went back to California to work it out with her much older husband. Which, time would show, failed miserably.

My grandparents had to scrounge to get everything they needed for a baby and had me for the next 6 months. They didn't hear back from my mother in all of that time. I can only imagine, from later in life experience, how difficult that entire ordeal must have been for my mother's family, but later on, when I got to meet them all, the bond that we would share started right there, when I was an infant.

My grandparents, as well as my two aunts and one uncle loved me, but I'm sure I was a burden on them. The kids were all teenagers, and my aunt, Michelle, grew the most attached to me. It was up to her to watch me during the day while my grandparents worked.

Michelle, at the age of 17, learned how to care for a baby, and her motherly instincts kicked in. She also used the time to take as many pictures of me as she could. Later, I would see albums of pictures of me as a baby with my grandparents and family. The ones with me and my grandfather were my favorites. He was a true rock star. Handsome and Irish, he had a very charming and convivial way about him. People loved my grandfather, but no one more than my grandmother. The love they shared, that I saw later in life, has stayed with me ever since.

Eventually, my father and my mother divorced, and my father got full custody of my brother and me, a feat that was amazing in the state of California in the late 1970s. Most mothers were given custody of the children in divorce proceedings, and I'm sure my father had to fight to get us back.

So, my mother flew to Boston to retrieve me, and take me back to California. When my aunt Michelle found out about this, she told her parents she wanted to take me on one last walk. They found her 6 miles away, running away with me. I can imagine her heartache. She didn't see me again for 26 years.

So, back to California I went.

I grew up not knowing any of what had happened in the first year of my life. Of course, Jasper had no memories of where he had been either. I'm not sure what became of my biological mother after she gave us to our father, but we had no contact with her until I was 7 and a half years old and my father was sick.

I don't want anyone to think that my biological mother did not love my brother and me, but she was beset on all sides by my father's family, who were all very powerful and influential where they were from.

My mother's family told me later in life that my biological mother felt ganged up on and she had to fight my father's family every day of their life together.

At the age of 40, I can now appreciate what she had gone through, and I only regret that I didn't get to know her as an adult. I imagine we would have had so very much in common. Including the history of fighting my father's family.

Looking back now, I can completely see and sympathize with my Wolff's family beliefs about my father. Margrit was only 20 years old when she met my father, who was over 50. In a lot of ways, he was a predator.

So, please see the wool that had been pulled over our eyes until we were adults about who my father really was, and which I'm going to write about further, from the mindset I had my entire life until the last year.

The truth of things didn't come to light until I was so despondent and in a dark place. I didn't realize through my life that my father's family caused so much of the mental anguish I lived with. From my father's own mouth when I was a baby, they believed I wasn't his. And that's ok. Since I found out the truth, I did the DNA testing online, and was connected to my father's family completely. So, joke's on them.

Because I'm a pretty awesome guy now, and they will never have a chance to know that.

I can only imagine what my mother, Margrit, had gone through with them.

So, in the meantime, my father, had fallen in love with my biological mother's college roommate, Linda. She became my stepmother and I grew up with her. Her and my father had two girls, within a year of each other.

Growing up, we had, what we thought, was a happy life.

There were four of us, my brother Jasper, me, and my two little sisters, Zoie, and Harmony.

I knew that we were poor, I just didn't know how poor. My father still gave sermons at our church, but he didn't work there full time. He worked as a handyman, a carpenter, and painter, picking up jobs where he could.

5

He supplemented his income with fishing the docks at 3am so we had dinner, and there were many times that we all piled into the station wagon and drove around town, to different grocery stores, and my dad would dumpster dive for extras. I still can't eat cantaloupe to this day because of finding them more than anything else in the dumpsters and eating around the rotten parts.

I didn't know how other people lived. But I knew that we weren't doing very well, very early on. My favorite memory was a Christmas that we were chosen to be a Salvation Army family. They brought toys and bikes for us all, and it was just the best Christmas. I didn't know it would be our last one as a family.

Linda had a son from a previous marriage. His name was Tony. He was a lot older than us and had a real chip on his shoulder. He was an extremely angry teenager. My father would work every day, and my mother couldn't handle us children very well, so she left it up to Tony to discipline us. He was especially heavy handed with me. I can remember quite clearly a few times of him punching me and throwing me up against walls until my teeth rattled. But the worse is when he burned my palms on the hot stove.

I stayed up all night with my hand in a cup of ice water, watching MTV with him. I can remember that happening twice. I don't know if my father knew what had happened, or if my mother and Tony covered it up and I was too afraid to tell my dad the truth, or if he knew, and did nothing. Either way, I grew up with a lot of fear. At that point, the fear was mostly physical.

My brother and I were rough boys and got into fights all the time. I have a couple of scars on the back of my head from different times it got busted open from being too rough.

And then, when I was 8 years old, my father found out that he had terminal pancreatic cancer. He was given less than a year to live and had to make some decisions. He had four children under the age of 9.

So, he contacted my biological mother and told her he was sending Jasper and I to her in New Jersey. It was her turn to be a parent.

So, having to say goodbye to the only family I knew, we got on a plane for the first time in our lives, so we thought, and flew to someone we did not know.

I remember so vividly meeting my biological mother and my new little sister and brother. Their father was not in the picture anymore but lived close by. He was not a good person at all. Drugs and violence and prison ruled his life. He scared the crap out of me, and later, when my mother knew that, she would send me to his trailer for punishment. He would threaten me with a huge hunting knife. He was a big guy as well, and I was little for my age.

Meeting my biological mother in that New Jersey airport was not a positive experience for me. She wanted me to call her Mom, but I could not do it. She was not my mother. It was a fight we would have for several more weeks, finally ending with me calling her mom, but grudgingly. I knew things were going to be bad when she asked us if we were hungry. She had split pea soup at home, which was so gross, I almost threw up.

We lived with my biological mother for two months. Over which was Christmas. I just remember that a lot of bad things happened because my mother could not handle all her children, and we were always a burden. I will describe one situation that happened so that you can see what it was like. But again, as an adult now, I can completely understand and accept her choices in life. She made the best decisions she could with what she had. I have had to do the same so

7

many times, it's impossible now for me to not forgive what my young mother had had to do.

My little sister, Venus Layne, and I got to be very close. We both looked just like my mother, so we were always called "the twins." We decided to run away from home one day and go back to my family in California. We took a five-dollar bill from my mother's purse and walked to the corner store to get provisions. In our very young minds, this meant chocolate candy bars. We each bought one Crunch Bar, and decided that what we really wanted was candy, and not to run away. So, we ate our chocolate bars, and went home.

My mother found out what we had done because you didn't lie to her. She was big and mean. She didn't punish my sister. But me, she went to the store and bought three big bags of leftover Halloween chocolate, and for the next two weeks, that was all I was allowed to eat, breakfast, lunch, and dinner. She even packed it for me to eat at school.

I would trade it for real food, because after two days of that, I threw up just smelling chocolate. That went on for two weeks. I don't know how long it would have lasted if the school didn't say something to her about me always bringing just candy for lunch.

My biological mother was constantly hospitalized for her strong bi-polar behavior and had to be heavily medicated. She was on lithium treatments, and we never knew which way she would be when she was home. Our solace was our babysitter. She was halfway normal.

After two months, she contacted my dying father and told him, with us standing there, that she didn't want us anymore. That she couldn't handle it.

My father sent plane tickets. Jasper was sent to Texas to live with my father's sister, Virginia. For some reason, I went back to California. By this time, my father and mother and little sisters didn't live in the house I grew up in anymore.

As the cancer progressed, he couldn't work. They were living in a two-bedroom apartment, two towns over from where I had grown up. My father had lost half of his considerable weight by this time.

My father was over 6 ft. 2 in when I was growing up. Even in his 50's and 60's he was a big, strong, man. But the man I saw at the airport back in California was almost the same size as me at the age of 8.

We went twice a week to get his abdomen pumped at the hospital. He would fill up with fluid and bile and they would pump gallons of it out of him. He would always stop at Kentucky Fried Chicken on these trips and get us kids Chicken Littles. Little chicken sandwiches they had in the 1980's.

As you can imagine, by this time, I started to have a fear of rejection and abandonment. This fear came to control my life until I was 40 years old. There are many more reasons for this, but it started right here. Saying goodbye to my family at the age of 8, and then my mother telling my dad that she didn't want me, all of this started the enemy whispering in my sub-conscious that I wasn't worth anything.

That voice got stronger and stronger as I got older.

Chapter 2

I'm now eight years old. My father was getting weaker by the day. He was the strength for all of us. He had been such a big presence throughout my early life. He kept everyone together. But he was about to die, and he knew it.

I know he was a strong Christian, but what prayers he must have been praying for his children! I like to think back that he did love and care for us, and wanted the best for us, but what could he do? He was about to die horribly at the young age of 63.

He had no control over anything. I can imagine he must have been in so much pain, physically and mentally. The only way he could have had peace is if God told him we would be taken care of. But as life progressed, there was very little of that for all four of us.

When my father got sick, I think the feeling around the family was that nothing was going to be the same. Linda was very codependent on my father. She looked to him for everything. I don't think she had ever been a very strong person. She was an obsessive over-eater. She was obese and had severe back problems because of it. After my father passed, she had to start using crutches and a walker, and never was able to get away from help with walking until the end of her short life.

When May came around, my father took a turn for the worse. He couldn't get out of bed, and the nurses had to come to him to remove the excessive fluid buildup in his abdomen and administer the pain medication that made him sleep more than anything else. I and my sister, Zoie, were still going to elementary school every day, but even the school knew that we would be called home at any time. During the last couple of weeks, I do not remember any family or friends coming around. There were no visitors, and for the first time in my life, I started feeling alone.

One night in particular stands out. I don't remember the day, or what was happening in my young world, but I remember hearing my father's voice call my name from his dark room. I hesitantly walked into the dismal, low lighted room, and saw his shrunken body under the blankets. He called me close and started talking to me.

To this day, I have no recollection of what he said, past the expected, "take care of your sisters and your mom" thing.

But I know in my heart that what he said next, and to which is lost in my mind and memories, hit me deep, and has stayed with me to this day. I like to think he imparted some wisdom, something which has made me a better man. I would like to think he told me he loved me.

I have no idea what he said. I don't know why I can remember everything else so sharply, too sharply sometimes, but I cannot remember the last thing my father said to me, as he lay dying.

I have gone back and forth with trying hypnosis to try to bring the memories back to the surface, but I really don't know how I feel about what I would learn, if there was anything more than the garbled words of a very sick man, at the end of his life. I may just try to find comfort in my delusions that it was something grand and wonderful. Something I can try to impart to my own children one day, made up from my imagination, but maybe with a kernel of truth that he told me that spring night.

I started acting out after this. That's normal, in such a stressful situation. I can remember one time, when the apartment pool opened, my sister and I went swimming, but had to promise to stay in the shallow end. I can still see myself, not knowing how to swim well at this time, walk over to the diving board at the deep end, and jump off to my sure death. But something incredible happened. Apparently, I needed to risk death to learn how to swim. I came to the surface of the water, took a deep breath, and swam back to the shallow end. From that day on, from some sub-conscious place, I was an excellent swimmer. But that was God's hand as well.

A few days later, at the same pool, my little sister Zoie was playing by the deep end, and one of the neighbor boys thought it would be funny to push her into the pool. I don't think he realized that she could not swim, and if he did, I hope he burns in hell. Anyway, I saw it all happening from some tables on the other side, and I don't think I ever ran faster in my life. I jumped in, and not being very big or strong, I was still able to save her. I pulled her over to the side, so she could reach out, and walk the side of the pool wall to the shallow side and get out. I know for a fact that if I had not done what I did a few days previously, I would not have been able to save her, and I would be less one wonderful, beautiful sister right now. Things would go on to get very, very bad for the two of us, but she reminds me, even today, that we were so close through all of it, for the trials to come, and she was always sad when they would take me away. I have forgotten a lot of what was to happen, but she hasn't. It's always a sobering conversation when we reminisce. I would be taken a world away, but I have to remember that she is still there, in the same neighborhood, and her ghosts are always present.

On the night of the 8th of May 1988, my father was taken by the paramedics, and ensconced into the ICU of the local hospital. We went to school

12

the next morning and had plans to go visit my father right after school. When we got home, my mother was preparing things to take to the hospital for an overnight stay. She received a phone call at around 4:30pm. It was the hospital staff giving her the update that my father had died in his sleep about an hour earlier. They told her that he just drifted away, with no one in the room, and the next nurse to come in to check his vitals found him gone. His official time of death was 3:50pm on May 9th, 1988. He was 63 years old.

My mother screamed into the phone and broke down crying. Zoie and I were in the courtyard below the apartment and heard the terrible scream. Zoie looked at me and said, "Daddy died."

It was difficult to see Linda react that way, as we all knew what was coming. I think that most of the grief came from the fact that when my father died, he was alone. It saddens me to this day to know that not one person in his family, nor one of his eight children, or any of his many friends were there to say goodbye as he slipped away. My faith tells me that he was not alone. That Jesus was right there with him, to guide him to paradise. But in life, he had been there for so many people, and not one of them were there with him at the end. My eight-year-old brain on that day felt shame for focusing on what I learned in school that day. I don't remember even thinking about my father that day. He was in so much pain, in ICU, alone and weak, and probably unconscious, but I didn't even think of him that day. I knew we were going to see him in the hospital that evening, but we had done that so many times in the last six months. I feel shame to this day that we weren't there. My logical brain knows that I couldn't have done anything as an eight-year-old. But I feel bad anyway.

We drove up to the hospital when my mother calmed down. We walked down the hallways we had walked down so many times before. The nurse led us to a room where my father's body still lay. We all shuffled in. My mother, my sisters, Tony, and me. There was a priest there, and I remember my mother, who was raised Catholic, prayed with him. My sisters and I walked up to the side of the bed and my father lay there with his eyes closed, not moving, and looking very gray. The sheet was pulled up to his neck, and I was waiting for his eyes to open and for him to look at me. To this day, I have the same feeling every time I see a dead body at a funeral. My imagination has them opening their eyes and turning their heads and looking right at me. I get the exact thought every single time.

My mother wanted us to say goodbye to our father but told us we would see him again at the funeral. We were not in that room for very long. By this time, my father's best friend, Morris, showed up with his wife, who we called Lou. Morris took Zoie and I, as well as a distraught Harmony, down to the cafeteria and got us cups of pudding. Harmony kept saying "Daddy is sleeping. We have to wake up Daddy."

Tony stayed with mom, and apparently, they were all planning for the funeral and burial. My father had been in the Navy early in life, and the arrangements for a military funeral were already in place. The funeral would be three days later. His Navy career wasn't something he spoke about to us children, but I would learn a lot about it later in life.

We went home, and I just remember having to go to school the next day. When my mother picked us up after school, we got a huge surprise. Jasper popped up in the back seat. I had not seen him since leaving New Jersey six months prior. We all hugged and laughed together. It was a bright spot in a dismal day. He had an early birthday present for me, as my birthday was three weeks away. I wasn't allowed to open it yet, but he told me it was a new Walkman. I was very excited, as I had gotten some new tapes recently.

The funeral was beautiful. All the people from my father's life were there, including his four oldest children. I had met them each once or twice in my life, but not enough to really know anything about them. I do know that my mother allowed my father's flag to be given to his oldest son, John. I thought that was very unfair at the time, but looking back now, I see the sacrifice my mother made for that.

I hope that John knows to this day how special that is, and that currently, my father's four youngest children have absolutely nothing of my father's. I have three pictures with him in them, and that is all I have of anything to do with my father. Anything that showed my father had been alive and in so many people's lives belongs to his oldest children, who had him for most of their own lives. I only had him for eight years, and those times are heavily clouded in lost memories from time going by.

I hope his older four children know what a blessing they must have had to have known him for so long, and for their mother to still be alive, even today. I have a lot of bitterness built up for my four oldest siblings, who, when everything went to crap for the four younger children, didn't do anything for us.

It wasn't our fault that our father made the decisions that he made.

I don't talk to the oldest four to this day because I feel like they don't deserve to know us. They probably don't care, but we have the same blood, and to some people, that means something.

I remember walking up to my father's body at the funeral. The song, "I'll Fly Away" was being sung. I just remember not crying.

People were telling me I should cry. I just couldn't. I felt bad for that.

The truth is, I didn't cry for my father's death until I was 39 years old. It took a very intense series of ETT sessions to get to that point. After that, I spent the next year crying at the drop of a hat. Like a floodgate opened. I had so much emotion built up from over thirty years of suppressed grief and anger.

The journey I have been on for over a year now started in the office of my therapist, who pointed out that there was a little boy who no one hugged, or talked to, or asked what he was feeling.

That little boy built up so many walls that he didn't know how to make any relationship work since then. That little boy turned into a man who made every bad decision he could, not knowing that it was because he had to get those emotions out.

That little boy never knew how to connect with another person because he lost everything he loved and couldn't process it correctly. The lies he believed about himself became a self-fulfilling prophesy that almost destroyed him thirty-two years later. The circumstances that happened after his father died made everything so much worse. The dirt being rubbed into those raw, un-healed wounds made it so that those wounds would not close for almost half a lifetime later.

How much could that little boy put up with in life? He was about to find out. He was about to find out hard.

Chapter 3

After my mother made us approach my father's body, laying in the plain, wooden casket, we were told to go outside the funeral home and play. I remember my father looking very gray. They had commented on how the funeral home had left his mustache, which apparently wasn't normal procedure. He had worn that thick mustache for most of his life, so it was fitting that he was buried with it. He looked more filled out then he had in the hospital the last time I saw him. My child brain didn't comprehend that the embalming process was used to make him look his best for the funeral. He was wearing his gray suit that he had worn to church so many Sundays. All in all, I wasn't afraid to see him. I felt bad because I wasn't crying. People were making comments about how it was ok for me to cry, but that just made me feel horrible that I wasn't crying.

The fact that I didn't cry would stick with me for many years, and when my aunt cornered me in her kitchen as a small for my age 11-year-old, years later, and was yelling at me to talk about how I was feeling, I just couldn't. I couldn't process what had happened to me at that time until I was 39 years old, and it was such a relief, I was able to sleep all the way through the night for the first time in at least 25 years. The mental release of all those emotions literally knocked me out.

My brother and two sisters went out to the front of the funeral home and played tag in the grass. It was a beautiful northern California late-spring day. The sun was shining, and I could hear the gospel songs being sung inside the funeral.

"Amazing Grace" led to "I'll Fly Away" once again, led to "the Old Rugged Cross". All my father's favorite old gospel. I still love listening to those old hymns. The Navy Honor Guard was there, getting ready to lead the procession to the burial site. When my mother came out and collected us, we were sweaty and happy, and were told to calm down and get ready to show proper respect at the grave site.

My father's grave was situated in the same part of the Bay Area where we had grown up in his church, in El Cerrito, at the top of the Albany Hills. We saw that after the procession of cars made it to the road next to the grave, you could look north while standing next to his headstone, and you would see the Golden Gate Bridge was suspended perfectly between two tall pine trees situated at the end of the cemetery road, where it ended in a turn-about. A lot of people commented on this phenomenon. It really was a beautiful sight. I have only visited my father's grave once since burying him. That same scene is still present. The bridge suspended between the two trees at the end of the cemetery road. I have thought long and hard about how I want to be taken care of when I die. I really do not want to be buried. At this stage in my life, I'm not married, and I don't have anyone that I would want to be buried next to, with no family history of a specific burial place. So, I would like to be cremated and my ashes scattered somewhere beautiful. Saying that, though, my father deserved as much of a beautiful burial place as possible, and the scene you see when you visit his grave, with the bridge off in the distance, suspended between the two tall, green, evenly spaced trees, along with the green grass and lovely, country smells, is quite the fitting place.

The Navy Honor Guard was doing the rifle salute, and the guns were going off, bringing me back to the present. We were supposed to each drop a white rose onto my father's simple casket as it was lowered into the ground. I was cognizant of my duties at this burial. I had a job required of me as one of his children. My mother whispered to us that it was time, and as the machine used to lower the casket started humming to life, we each walked to the edge and dropped in the rose that someone had handed to us when we walked up to the hole in the ground.

I stood at the edge of the grave, looking down at the closed casket slowly descending into the ground. I don't think I was even thinking anything at the moment. The feeling I felt, as that eight-year-old boy was an overwhelming feeling of being lost.

Everything was changing. Jasper was returning to Texas the next day. I didn't know when I would see my brother again. I wondered what we would have for lunch. I'm sure there were many child-like thoughts running through my mind at that minute.

My mother was behind me whispering for me to hurry. Other's wanted a turn at the grave. I dropped in my rose, and it didn't stay on top of the casket. It fell between the casket and the side of the grave so that I'm sure the casket landed on it, crushing it.

I was upset about that. My brother's and sister's roses were on top of the descending casket. Mine was lost to the grave. I felt sad. I also started to feel anger. In just a couple of short months, that anger would be all that I felt.

I moved back to my seat where my brother wanted to talk about where the roses landed. I wanted to watch the Honor Guard fold the flag that had been draped across my father's coffin. After folding it, and re-folding it, making it into a very tight triangle, they walked over, and presented it to my oldest brother, John.

I looked at my mother and she was crying. To this day, I don't know why she made the choice for the flag to be given to my father's oldest child. I think it was to keep the peace, but I also think it was an admission of guilt for having been with my father when he should have been with his first family.

How utterly unfair that the older children couldn't or wouldn't have anything to do with our family as we were growing up. I could have had so much more family, and this would become so glaringly obvious to me in the memories ahead where I was so utterly alone.

I'm sure, when I think of it logically, that they had their own problems and ideas about my father's choices. But they took that out on us children.

Later in life, when social media was such a big thing, my older brother Mike would reach out. I was congenial, but very distant. The other three never tried. Their loss.

Going back home after the funeral, I just remembered wanting to get out of the Sunday clothes I was in. My child's mind just wanted to hold on to anything that resembled normalcy. So, we all went down to the play area and played again.

I remember always being told to go play a lot as a child. We were always excluded from the adult's conversations. I think the adults would do that to protect the children, but also, because they had an idea that children should be seen and not heard.

As a father, I always tried to include my children into discussions, but also made boundaries they were expected to follow. When two adults were talking, they didn't interrupt. I don't really know the "why" you should treat children in this regard, but I know as a child, it was better that we were outside playing then being underfoot.

The next three weeks went by without much notice. We were getting close to summer break. My brother Jasper flew back to Texas. We spoke on the phone a couple of times, but that came less and less as the days went by. I remember being a little excited about my birthday coming up, but my mom was so stressed out that all she had to live off was the social security checks that started coming in the mail every month. My 9th birthday came and went with only one difference.

Obviously, my father wasn't there, so my mother wanted to change things up a bit. Instead of the chocolate cake she always made for my birthday, she asked me if I wanted a different choice.

I loved cheesecake, so told her I would like a cheesecake. She sent Tony to the store and he came back with a round, strawberry covered cheesecake for my birthday.

Three weeks after we buried my father, I was looking at this cheesecake for my birthday, without candles to blow out, and only being enjoyed by my sisters Zoie and Harmony, me, my brother Tony, and my mom.

It was more of a somber moment than anything. I think I went to bed early.

It was just too sad to enjoy.

Chapter 4

The next three months went by rather quickly. I'm expounding on these times in my life because they really shaped who I would be for the next 30 years.

Two things during that summer after we buried my father stand out. The first, is that before my birthday, at the beginning of June, my mother started dating again. She started using 1-900 numbers, as that was the dating venue of the late 80's.

I distinctly remember two of the guys she brought around that summer. The first guy, I think his name was Bob, took me and my sister to the drive-in movies to see Who Framed Roger Rabbit, which had just come out, and which we really wanted to see. I don't remember my mother going with us to this movie, which makes me think that she brought a guy into our lives, very quickly after my father passed away, and gave him permission to take her children to the movies without her. Looking back now, that is such dangerous behavior. I don't think Bob lasted very long, because then my mother met Louie.

Louie was the opposite of my father.

He was loud, and very abusive. He was a drinker, and there was a lot of concern that he was using my mother's social security money to buy drugs.

My brother Tony did not like him, and as Louie was around more and more, Tony finally moved out on his own, and never came back. He eventually had a son and became a very responsible and loving father. I think his son, Dylan, changed his life.

Louie did not like my mother having children. That was very apparent early on. He was controlling and had a very bad temper. My adult experience shows me that my mother kept him around because of father-figure issues that she had. Louie was a lot older than her, as my father had been. I know she was a very co-dependent person, who clung to any man that showed her attention, as well as dominated her life. Like I had alluded to earlier, she was not a strong person. I loved her tremendously, but she made a lot of bad choices.

At the end of July, after Louie had been in our lives for a month or so, somehow, he convinced my mother that I needed to be in a nearby boy's home for my own good. It was a Catholic boy's home, financed by the state, and had very strict rules. My mother conceded and took me to have an interview with the acceptance office.

I remember being in this office with an older man and he was asking me questions about how much I would get into trouble, if I got into fights, and if I wanted to live in the boy's home.

I won't name the place, but anyone in Northern California is sure to know the place I'm describing. It's still there, and still running strong.

My mother used the fact that my father had just died, and I had run away from home a couple of times when I was younger to get the boys home to accept me. A few weeks later, I was driven from my home, said goodbye to my mother and little sister once again, and given over to the care of the home for troublemaking boys in Northern California.

When they walked me into my dormitory, where 17 other boys lived, I felt real shame for the first time in my young life. I had all my belongings in a brown paper Safeway bag. I had two shirts, two pairs of jeans, and some socks

23

J.L. Fox | I Won't Be Shaken

and underwear. No toys, no belongings, nothing that most of the other boys had. When I was shown into my room I shared with two other boys, they both had posters on the walls, drawers filled with toys and gadgets and belongings. I had two shirts, two pairs of jeans, some run down tennis shoes, and some underwear. I finally saw just how poor I was. I was ashamed of myself, and my life. Not to mention, I was once again given away, thrown away, and not wanted. This seemed to become a theme in my life. I cried the first night I was in the boy's home. I was alone. Truly alone.

The first month at the boy's home was ruled by school, and activities. They promoted sports, church, communal gathering for meals, and work. We all had chores, and we were expected to keep everything clean. Every Wednesday night, every dormitory would turn on the television for a movie that was played from the head office. I remember they would ask what the movie would be every week, and the man in charge would always have the same answer. "Gandhi" he would say.

One week, it was "Gandhi" and that was the funniest thing that I think had ever happened in my life.

Another, amazing experience at that time stands out. I started reading. I started reading a lot. I lost myself in books like The Hardy Boys, and adventure books like "My Side of the Mountain", "Hatchet" and mysteries by Joan Lowry Nixon and Mary Higgins Clark. I read Tolkien and got into reading Choose your Own Adventure books. I remember most everything that happened at the boy's home, but these two things stand out the strongest in my memories.

My insatiable appetite for books, and the things that started happening at nighttime.

The nighttime activities would shape who I became as an adult more than anything else besides losing my father. For almost four weeks, circumstances would take place that made me question everything about myself and God, as well as causing the curtain to be pulled back from my young eyes and I saw what this world really all was about.

There were two older boys in my room in the dormitory in which I lived.

I remember they were 14 and 15, respectably. I was nine years old at this time, and as I look at my daughter today, who is nine years old, I can't imagine her ever going through what I went through. She's an amazingly intelligent and able child. But she is a child first and foremost. She hasn't had the easiest life either, but I look at her and envision myself at the same age.

I was, again, little for my age, and was very innocent and gullible. I was poor and given to bouts of anger and depression. For these kinds of teenage boys, I was an amazingly easy target, and grudgingly obedient in what they ended up doing to me.

After I had been at the boy's home for about two months, the two teenage boys in my room started sexually abusing me. It started out slowly. They groomed me over a period of about three weeks. It started with small things. Asking me to touch them. Telling me about masturbation, and how good it felt. I was made to watch them masturbate together late at night.

I could feel my own body responding, but I always felt dirty about it.

Sexualization of young children matures them very quickly. I had no experience with these things in my short nine years of life. So, in a way, it was exciting, and made me look complacent in what happened. I felt guilt for these things for a very long time. It wasn't until a therapist made it clear that at nine years old, I did not have the capacity to take credit for what eventually started happening.

After a short time, the sexualization turned into rape. Every single night I was eventually made to use my mouth, and then my body, in very painful ways

25

for the pleasure of these two boys. I don't think any of the other boys in the home knew about it, but in my mind, everyone knew.

I felt shame, remorse, displeasure, pain, and finally an overwhelming guilt. The nightly rapes would last for about four weeks before I told an adult about it. It hurt every single time.

I bled and was made to feel like I had to enjoy it and that I did enjoy it because my body would respond in a way that made the teenagers think I enjoyed it. I questioned my own sexuality even when I didn't know what that meant. Was I gay? Did I like boys? I grew up right outside San Francisco, where being gay wasn't as socially unaccepted as in some other parts of the country at that time.

It became four weeks of nightly torture, which I had to put a stop to. So, I did what the catholic priests had been telling me to do for three months. I went to confession.

At confession, I told the priest everything that had happened, and he asked me a lot of very specific questions. I named the two boys who had been doing this to me and gave him all the details he asked for. He kept telling me I needed to purge all the sins out of my life if I was to be forgiven. I believed these things. At the end of the confession, he made me feel that what had happened was my fault for allowing it to go on, and that I had confessed to liking some of the feelings it gave me. I didn't know that in a lot of rape cases, the victim's body will show signs of arousal, without them being aroused. This has made the rapist think that the victim is enjoying what is happening, rather than the opposite being true.

I was given penitence by the priest, seven Hail Mary's and four Our Father's, and the next day, I was moved out of the dormitory I had lived in. I don't know if the teenage boys were punished for what happened to me. I never saw either of them again. No one at the boys home ever said anything more to me about it, and I feel like it was swept under the rug, and I was given no chance to heal from it. It was never mentioned again, and I felt like I couldn't tell anyone else. I never told my mom, or later my aunt and uncle about what happened. I didn't tell my brother Jasper what had happened until less than a year ago. I didn't completely heal from these things for many years. I just couldn't talk about these things to anyone. My first wife didn't know about these things. I was able to tell my second wife about them, but it turned into an unhealthy conversation between us, and I felt judged for the situation. I finally received support for these things, and healing, and the ability to talk about it.

The nightly rapes, and the abuse of my body, and my spirit, and my innocence gave me an uncommon dislike for myself. I felt shame after these things happened. Even as an adult, shame connected with sex would hamper any healthy relationship I tried to make. At the age of nine I started to masturbate. I had become sexualized at that young age, and it was extremely unfair.

The thing that hurt the most, is that in all of this, I felt such a keen understanding that losing my father caused all these things.

Being thrown away by my mother once again for the sake of her new boyfriend, being alone, and the abuse I went through was all God's fault for taking my father from me.

The anger was now a boiling rage inside of me that I couldn't get out. That rage would grow in me, and would come out against people who loved me, and who I was incapable of loving in return. I did not have the room in my heart to love, because it was filled with this all-consuming pain and anger.

And during all this turmoil inside of me, I still didn't have an adult who was there to just hug me, try to understand me, or to give me reassurances like my father had done for me most of my life. All this pain and anger was overshadowed with a huge sense of loneliness. I felt so damn alone. I remember that feeling more than any other from this time in my life.

Chapter 5

After being at the Catholic boy's home in Northern California for a year and a month, my mother came and picked me up one day. I'm not sure what caused her to come get me, but I really appreciated it. I did not like the boy's home, but I did like the opportunities I had there. I was growing, becoming better at sports, and especially swimming. I made some friends but didn't keep up with them after I left. There was one more benefit that I was learning that would shape my life. My introduction to very early computers. We were playing games like "Oregon Trail" and I was, early on, very proficient with the use of these computers. I really enjoyed the technology and would later have jobs that gave me access to learning as much about things like coding, and writing, as well as other programming experience with these computers. I loved the technology.

After my mother picked me up the next summer, I was 10. I was still little for my age, but I had grown a bit awkwardly. I was getting taller but was still very much a child. She took me to the small efficiency she lived in with Zoie and Louie.

Harmony had been put in foster care while I was in the boy's home, but there was word that the family she lived with in Lodi, CA may want to adopt her. She was originally taken away from my mother because she was suicidal. Linda was always so very abusive towards Harmony. Looking back now, Zoie and I remark how it seemed like Harmony was not around during all this time, but she was. Linda kept her isolated, and she missed my father so much. She was

29

convinced that he was just asleep. She tried to commit suicide at a very young age. She has had to go through some of the worse of all of this. Her strength as an adult is a testimony to her drive and compassion, and overwhelming spirituality. I marvel at all of my siblings, but Harmony has truly risen above her childhood.

I'm not sure how my mother felt about her being adopted, but I do remember going and visiting Harmony, who seemed just as sad and little as she always did. I wasn't that close to Harmony, and I'm still not. She has become a teacher for other children that grew up how she had grown up. She is very successful at JobCorp and gives of herself more than anyone else I've ever known. I don't know that she has a fulfilled life now, as she has never married or had children, but she is amazingly spiritual, and has such a close relationship with God. I know we were all affected by our upbringing, and I know it shows in our adult lives, but she has maintained that spiritual connection through it all and is stronger than anyone else I know. I know she has gone through a lot of the same things I have, but I think, in a lot of ways, she is so much stronger than I am. I don't talk to her much now, but I know where she is, and I hope she knows I will always be here for her.

Likewise, Zoie is a teacher. A couple of years after my father passed away, she was also put into the California foster care system, but she was adopted by a pastor who was close friends with my father, after her own stint in a group home. She doesn't talk much about that time of her life, but looking at her as an adult, she is obviously affected by it, and also, like Harmony, perseveres past what the statistics says she should.

She grew up with that amazing family in the same neighborhood we had lived in before my father got sick. She hasn't left the area in all this time. She is the closest to what and where we lived while my father was alive. But she, too, has never been married or had children. She gives so much of herself to those she loves. I, again, know we are all affected by these events, but my sisters have shown a strength I just don't possess. They are amazing, strong women. I cherish them very much.

I stayed with my mom, Louie, and my sister in the apartment in Hayward, CA for a very short time. Soon after, we moved to an even smaller apartment behind a bar that was owned by my mom's best friend and her husband, on San Pablo Blvd, in San Pablo, CA. The worse section of the Bay Area, besides Oakland. The neighborhood was rife with gang activity, homelessness, and extreme poverty. My mother was still receiving the Social Security checks for me, and my sister, as well as survivor's benefits for herself. Louie was using this money to supply his habits. We did not eat well, and did not have good clothes, or hygiene. My mother forgot how to be a mother. She was disabled, extremely overweight, and very deponent on her children doing everything for her. Many times, I was called home from school to do something as benign as set up the Nintendo for her, so she could play from her bed.

In the evenings, Zoie and I were made to go to bed early, and we would listen to Louie and my mother having sex. He would then leave to go to the bar, and later in the night, my mom would wake me up to go into the bar and make Louie come home. He would always be drunkenly abusive, hitting me, and trying to get me to fight him. I can remember one time being so angry that I did push him away, which caused him to stumble in our living room, and he got up with an enraged, red face, and punched me so hard in the side of the head that I passed out. I did everything I could to be in the way from him hitting my sister. There was no way that was going to happen. But it did. I was powerless to stop a grown man from abusing us the way he would go on to do, but I tried my best.

There were so many bad situations at this time. I really don't want to go into them all, but I will touch on a couple, just to show the stark differences between our lives when my father was alive, and where we were afterwards.

One day, my mother had me go to the grocery store and get stuff for dinner. The actual food I was trying to cook alludes me, but I was a 10-year-old boy trying his best. I left a kitchen towel on the stove, and it caught fire. I tried to pick it up, fully ablaze, and it fell behind the stove. Zoie immediately started filling a pot with water and I grabbed the phone and called the fire department. We were resourceful if nothing else. After the hubbub died down, and the fire was extinguished, I think "those who be" started noticing the situation going on in that apartment. Later, things got to be very bad. While Linda was in the shower, and Zoie was helping her bathe, I remember hearing a small scream. I didn't find out until years later that in the shower, Linda had miscarried Louie's child. Zoie had to take the remains and flush it all down the toilet. The memory of that still haunts her. She told me recently that when she thinks of that time, she just remembers that it was her sibling that she disposed of. Again, her ghosts don't live very far from her.

Another situation that happened was even more disturbing. One evening, after school, Louie got my mom high on something. They thought it would be funny to try their hands at a little torture, as they put it. Louie started beating me with a belt, for no reason at all, while Zoie stood there in fear, watching. They were recording the sounds on a tape recorder. When he was done with me, he turned to Zoie. But Zoie was a screamer. He looked at her and said, "It's your turn." She started screaming like she had never screamed before. That was also on the tape. She fell to the ground, curled into a ball, and pleaded for him not to hit her. They both started laughing. Linda then took the tape to the bar owned by her best friend and started playing it. I found out later that her best friend, Fina, was so angry, she threw them both out, and did everything she could after that to watch out for Zoie and me.

One last memory comes to mind of the time in that small, dank, poverty-stricken apartment. Linda had been put into the hospital for a reason that we cannot remember. We just knew that she was the only thing keeping Louie in check when it came to us kids. Zoie and I went to school that day she was in the hospital, and we didn't want to go home. Zoie had a teacher named Ms. Costa, and she allowed us both to stay in her classroom until almost dark, cleaning the chalkboards and helping clean the classroom. I have no idea what those teachers all thought, but I knew that we were not the only cases of child abuse at that school. Reading books later in life, like "A Boy Called It," would show me that those times, in that area, were especially hard on children. And that's putting it lightly.

When we got home, later than usual, Louie had been drinking and wasn't very happy. He took his belt to us both, and I can vividly remember the imprint of that belt buckle on Zoie's legs. I don't think she wore a dress after that.

The next day, I was sent up to the hospital to stay with my mom. I remember a few things about that day. I remember how the nurses would say that I was a great son for spending time with my mom, and one brought me a GameBoy to play. I remember the bad food and thinking that my mom was going to die as well. But what I really remember is finding out that the hospital she was staying in just happened to be the hospital on my birth certificate. Alta Bates Hospital in Berkeley, CA. I walked up to the labor and delivery floor, because I had mentioned to a nurse that I had been born in this hospital. She told me that the walls outside the L&D wing was painted with all the names of the babies who had been born there, going back decades. I went up to it, checked the date of my birth, and did not see my name. It wasn't there. I have no idea why it wasn't there, but I remember feeling, not for the first time, like a failure in life. One more kick to the teeth, like so many others at this time.

I don't know why the school never said anything about the bruises and cuts on our faces and bodies, but they didn't. The one time that the school called the police and I was taken to the hospital was when my mom had me take one of her muscle relaxers before school so that I would "calm down". I was drugged throughout first period and the school took steps to find out what happened. This was the turning point that made the state of California respond to my father's last will and testament, which, I found out later, gave custody of Jasper and I to his two sisters who lived in Texas.

Not everything was horrible at this time, however. I know now that abuse and early adverse experiences would affect my health, both physical and mental later in life, but there was still blessings. One such, when I think back, was my sister and mine plan to get on the show, "Star Search." We made up a dance routine, practiced it every day, and knew that Ed McMann would pick us to win the 100-grand prize, and we would talk about how were would spend the money when we were rich. That dream, early on, gave me hope. It was a lesson I would use the rest of my life. No matter how bad things were to get, I would always hold onto dreams and hope, and use that to get through the adversity. I still do it to this day. I would do it a lot, as I was sent to live with a new family in Texas.

Once again, in my short life, I was saying goodbye to my family, and this time I was put on a plane for Texas. Right before this happened, the great earthquake of 1989 took place. I remember watching the World Series between the San Francisco Giants, and the Oakland A's, when the earthquake struck. It was 15 seconds of extreme fear for all Northern California. The bridges shook like a giant baby was using them for a rattle, and there was a two-decker freeway through Oakland that collapsed, killing a lot of people. As we drove to the San

Francisco Airport for my flight to a new life, we passed under that overpass. I looked up at the devastation made by a natural disaster of such magnitude and felt that I should have been under all that rubble and crushed concrete.

I had been given a white suit to wear by my mom's best friends, who had a son my age. It was short on my growing body, but I had to make a good first impression on the Texas relatives I had never met before.

Once again, I was being thrown away from my mom and sister, and everything that had anything to do with my father. In two short years, my life was unexpectedly upheaved, and I had a keen feeling that it was, again, God's fault. I didn't know how to pray to him, but I knew that I had no reason to. He wasn't powerful enough to bring back my dad, and obviously didn't care what had happened, and was continuously happening to a little for his age, nerdy, eleven-year-old boy. Off I went to a place I had never been before, but where my long-lost brother lived, but I would at least get to see Jasper again. On the plane, I ordered a ginger ale. My brother and I had been given ginger ale the first time we had flown out to New Jersey, and it seemed that was such a big thing in my short life. The only time in my short life that I had ginger ale seemed to be on airplanes, and to this day, I still order the same thing, every time I fly. That little cup of ginger ale is the only positive thing I can remember about this time of my life.

How sad is that?

Chapter 6

The cultural shock of moving from Northern California, in the worse, ghetto parts of the Bay Area, and growing up with such a mix of nationalities and cultures, to the Texas panhandle was unnerving. As the pilot called over the intercom of the plane that we were descending into the Lubbock International airport, I excitedly looked out the window. All I saw were cotton fields, and I had this overwhelming belief that we were going to land in hard packed dirt. I panicked for a second, wondering how we were going to make it if we had to bounce our way to a stop in a cotton field. I thought Texas was so backwards, that they didn't have a concrete runway, and that we had to land in the dirt. Every time I fly into Preston International Airport in Lubbock, TX, I look out the window and feel the same feelings and think the same things. Every time.

I got off the airplane and there was my brother standing next to a man I had never met. My brother and I hugged each other fiercely. I had not seen him in over two years. I remember running through the airport, racing each other, allowing that brotherly competition to burn through us. It still, to this day, burns through us. He is my closest family, and I have always depended on him, and him on me. As I write this, I will be having dinner with him tonight, and staying with him as my life slowly unfolds in where it is going today.

The man at the airport was my uncle Travis. He was the husband of my father's next oldest sister, Virginia, or Jenny, as well called her. Travis was a very short, skinny man who perpetually wore white collared shirts and dark slacks. I thought he was a travelling salesman from another era. Thick, prismed glasses perched on a sharp nose and disapproving glare stared back at me as Jasper and I ran ahead through the terminal, to see once again who was fastest.

Jenny and Travis were extremely spiritual. They attended an evangelical church that for the first time in my life, I saw the laying on of hands, as well as speaking in tongues, and people going into fits and shocks during services. As a child whose only experience with church was strict Baptist worship, and a year of Catholic services, this kind of extreme Christianity was shocking.

The house my brother had spent almost three years in, with Jenny and Travis, was not my destination.

My father had, in his cancer-riddled thought processes, given custody of me to his baby sister, Emily, or who we called, jokingly, Aunty Em, who lived in Amarillo, Texas.

Amarillo, I learned, was two hours to the north of Lubbock. I stayed with my brother for two weeks, until Jenny made me say goodbye to him, and drove me to my new home in Amarillo, with people I had never met.

I was extremely nervous.

But these family members, I learned, lived better than how I had grown up. They weren't poor, and never gave thought to just surviving. They were upper middle class.

When we pulled up to the modest home my new aunt and uncle lived in, I thought they were the richest people I had ever met. How does a kid go from living in a one-bedroom apartment on the back end of a bar covered in trash and poverty, to now live in a ranch style home with four bedrooms, and enough to eat every day? The cultural shock made me act out in ways that wasn't in character.

37

One instance from early on living with Emily, and my uncle Jerold, comes to mind.

One Sunday night, when the youth group at our church was finished, the church van was taking us all home. I begged and pleaded to be taken home first, which was way out of the way. They allowed this, and it was because I wanted all the other kids to see my house. I look at that house now as an adult and realized that I have owned larger and nicer houses than that one.

But I really wanted to show off how rich we were that night with the youth group. They, obviously, didn't care, but I was proud.

I was in the fifth grade when I went to live with Emily and Jerold. Within the first month of living there, I had the chicken pox. I then got staph infection on my face. I had the flu and broke an arm.

I can only assume how much of a burden I was on these people who were in their 50's and their three children were all grown and moved away and had families of their own.

I was also at an age that I needed a lot of support about changes in my body, and impressionable people in my life were giving me peer pressure to try things like alcohol and smoking. I didn't do these things, and obviously had never taken any drugs, but I could tell that my innocent aunt and uncle were at a loss on how to deal with a kid who was traumatized, came from a very inner-city rough neighborhood, and had things happen to him that he didn't talk about. And the fact that he lost all his family, and the life he knew, all before the age of 10.

I was bitter for a long time for the things my aunt and uncle later did with me, but looking back now, I know that they were out of their element. They tried their best. They took me to a child psychologist, but it was a waste of time and money because I was unable to open up and speak about the trauma in my young life.

When anyone tried to get me to talk, especially my aunt, I shut down hard and fast. She was about my size at this time, and I remember her cornering me in the kitchen after it had come to a head with the therapist and was screaming at me to talk to her. To tell her how I felt. She must had been so frustrated with me. I didn't even cry. I couldn't. I was so shut in in my feelings that they became a shield.

I used the anger and hurt to keep anyone else from hurting me. I was 11 years old and had built up walls that couldn't be penetrated. I had been thrown away so many times by now that I expected it from everyone. And as the next twenty years would prove, I was always right. Time and again, I was right. There must have been something so revolting about me that people who said they loved me would leave me sooner or later.

Relationships would come and go and always end the same way. I was made to feel never good enough. I was looking at fallen people in a fallen world for my sense of belonging and acceptance so many times, and was let down, so many times. I never looked to my heavenly Father for that acceptance, which He gives completely, and always, and never forsakes it.

It's still hard, at 40 years of age, to believe that fact.

Living with Emily and Jerold was both amazing and extremely life changing. Jerold was a large, quiet man with an amazing sense of humor. He was almost 100% Choctaw Indian.

He worked as an electrician for an oil company and was instrumental in developing their cryogenic processes. He was wicked smart, and wasn't keen on physical affection, other than wrestling and cajoling an impressionable young kid.

I loved Jerold fiercely because he reminded me so much of my father.

Jerold taught me the differences in hand tools as I would run back and forth from his shed in the back yard to the garage where he was perpetually working on one car or another. I would hold the flashlight for him and have to concentrate on where the beam shone so that he could see what he was doing. I was learning how to be a man and I didn't even realize it.

Jerold was always full of practical advice, and really demonstrated to me how to carry myself and respect myself. He taught me that my word was all I had. He taught me to be honest always and give back every chance I had.

He helped lead the music at church and had a powerful, southern singing voice. Thinking back now, knowing that I haven't spoken to my aunt and uncle for over 14 years, I miss Jerold the most, and still feel shame in the fact that I let him down.

I like to think, deep down, that he knows I am just doing my best.

Life is hard. He taught me to look it in the eye, and keep going, no matter what. I think that between my uncle and my father, I am the man that I am today. After all the mistakes, and selfish decisions, I hope they know that I have tried my hardest to live up to what they would want for me. I have tried to be the man they taught me to be. It's taken some time, but I am proud of the man I am today, because I was fashioned after these men.

Emily and Jerold encouraged me to get a job throwing papers on a paper route for my own money. They showed me the value of working for what I wanted, and not expecting it to be handed to me. If I wanted something, I worked for it. They were very heavy handed with discipline, but I think I needed a lot of that.

Like I said, and I want to reiterate, my uncle has always been one of the greatest men I've known. We had a falling out, and from my end, it was because my aunt made it very apparent that she had always felt like I wasn't my father's biological child.

Jasper looks just like my father. He has the same middle name as my father, the name that the family always called my father, because he had the same first name as his father. So, to my aunt, it was always a lot easier to accept my brother, and help him, then it was for me, who didn't look anything like my father.

I favor my mother completely and look just like her family. My father's family had always believed that my mother was a cheater and took advantage of my father. I didn't favor my father's family's looks. I was taller, darker, and skinnier. For this, my father's family has always shunted me some.

Later in life, I did the Ancestry DNA test. I was linked by my DNA to everyone else in my father's family that had done it.

I was obviously from my father and take more pride in my last name then most people in my family, because I was brought up to doubt where I came from. This was just another form of being thought of as not good enough, and I really want to take the results of the test, send them to the whole family with a big picture of a middle finger standing at attention.

I AM my father's son. It doesn't matter what I look like. I am proud of where I come from, even if that family treated me the way they did.

There were many more experiences living with Emily and Jerold. Their children, two boys and a girl, were close to me from the start. I loved my cousins very much.

Their oldest son, Terrance, had the same sense of humor as my uncle. I didn't know him very well, but his children were close to me until I left my aunt and uncle's house.

Emily and Jerold's middle son, Glen, was always a father figure to me. He was married to Rebecca, and the two of them were the perfect parents in my eyes. I would have given anything to live with them.

They eventually divorced but were such an amazing couple to an 11-year-old boy. They lived in Amarillo, really close by, while I lived with Emily and Jerold. I loved them so much. They were such a bright light in my dark life.

They, of course, were not aware of the things I had gone through, but I think they could sense that I had a rough childhood. They were amazingly patient with me and gave forgiveness easily when I ever did anything wrong. Their values and love held me up in a rough time of my life.

When I was a young adult, and going through even harder times, they were still always fun to visit and just have an easy, comfortable time with.

Glen also had an amazing sense of humor. He, more than anyone else, I thought, looked like me. He was tall and skinny and always had a busy air about him. He loved to work with his hands. He was always fixing things, and even did this for a living. He had an ability to look at a piece of machinery and just know how it worked. He could fix anything and had a rare talent for it.

He was what I wanted to be. He fixed things. There was nothing he couldn't fix. I respected that as a young boy more than anything, and it led me to have the career that I had.

His father, my uncle Jerold, was also a fixer of things. These men showed me that the truest form of being a man was being a man who could be depended on to fix things. And not just machines, or automobiles, or for me, airplanes.

But to fix their families. To be the backbone, and work with your spouse to get through life with a joke, and good humor.

Their example is something that I strive for. I hope that they read these words and know that I saw them for what they were. And what they were, were heroes to a broken little boy.

I can still hear their laughs and remember how they would wrestle with me as a boy, because they knew I needed that. I had lost my father very young, and I needed strong men in my life. More than anything, I needed the consistent love of a family man who had decided to take care of their families the best they could, and knew how to fix everything around them.

I have always been proud of the fact that my own children know that if anything, I am the man who fixes things for them. I couldn't fix the dark things in my mind and heart, but I could fix a car, or a toy, or a skinned knee.

I've been a poor example so many times in my life, but I have those early memories of the men put into my life to show me what I can strive to achieve. I see God in their examples.

Two of my better memories from living with Emily and Jerold were the Indian Powwows and rock collecting.

Jerold was almost full Choctaw Indian, as I've stated earlier. I learned about the Trail of Tears from him. He had full privileges from his heritage with the government, as did his children and grandchildren.

In Amarillo every year, they would put on an Indian Powwow. There would be hundreds of Native Americans dressed in full--historically accurate-- headgear and period dress.

I loved it. In the evenings, in a huge auditorium they would hold the circle dancing. A group of older members of the tribes represented would sit around the giant base drum and pound out the beat for the dancers.

Jasper and I went to one in particular and danced around the drumming circle for a very long time. Jerold took video of the dancing, and I can still remember years later watching it, and laughing at the pre-pubescent boys dancing with the beautifully arrayed Native Americans, wearing our jean shorts and hyper-color tee shirts, and around our waists, the notorious fanny packs bouncing around. We gyrated our skinny legs and flung our arms out with wild abandon. There was never more freedom in our young lives, and there has never been anything funnier seen on the planet in the history of funny sights than two nerdy white boys dancing with all that beauty around them and feeling the wild abandon of letting themselves go.

While we were at the Powwow, we shopped for artifacts and tourist souvenirs. Among the many things for sale were tables of polished rocks and semi-precious stones. Our eyes alighted on the dogs-tooth amethysts. My aunt bought us each one, and that night began my love for polishing rocks and finding geodes in the canyon close to Amarillo. The colors and beauty of the stones caught my attention and delighted me.

In a mundane, mostly brown landscape like the Texas Panhandle, finding a non-descript brown stone that when broken open reveals the beauty and wonder of a universe of color and brilliance gave my young imagination a world to become enamored with.

To this day I love amethysts and many other polished gemstones. Later, I would share that love with my children when we visited the Museum of Natural History in Washington, DC, and they would comment on how my eyes would light up at the beauty of this natural world.

After I had lived with Emily and Jerold for a little over a year and a half, they made a final decision concerning me.

At Labor Day, they took me out, 36 miles northwest of Amarillo, to Cal Farley's Boys Ranch.

During Labor Day weekend, Boys Ranch puts on their Annual Rodeo, and it was to that rodeo that they took me. My very first rodeo.

I was hugely excited but didn't know the real reason they took me out there. After watching the bull riding, the bronc riding, barrel racing, and pole bending, they asked me some very pointed questions on the ride home.

Did I like the place I visited? I had been in a boy's home before, was this one better? What was my opinion about the facts I learned about the place? And then the big one: would I like to live there?

I saw where this was headed. It had happened before. I remembered back to those same questions about the boy's home in California.

Here we go again, I thought.

I remember resigning myself to the fact that they didn't want me either. Here they were, giving me up, and only a few months since we had all gone to the courthouse in Lubbock, Texas, where my two aunts had legally adopted Jasper and me.

I felt like I knew the reason they adopted me. So, they could legally sign rights of me over to Boys Ranch. This one hurt the most since my father passed away.

I wanted nothing more in life than to be their child. I wanted Glen and Terrance, and their daughter Gina to be my siblings, who this time, if someone died, would take me in and take care of me.

I craved the safety of their family and wanted to be complete; a real part of it.

But no, it wasn't to be.

45

They couldn't handle me. They couldn't love me unconditionally and try as long as it took to get through to me.

How much was I at fault for not being able to be a perfect child for them, so they would keep me and love me, and raise me to be as happy as they all were?

How was I ever going to have the sense of humor and happiness that I saw in Glen and Rebecca?

So, I told them that it looked neat. I told them that I wouldn't mind going out there. I asked if they would come visit me.

I was so hurt inside by this, but the walls allowed me to say what they needed to hear to feel better about sending me to yet another boy's home. They justified it by saying that they weren't good for me, but they didn't try.

I'm sure in their minds they did the best they could. But as the next five years would prove, they drew further and further away, while expecting me to follow their guidance after graduating.

They gave up their rights to parent me with the choice to throw me away, yet again. I honestly don't think that they meant anything bad by it. I obviously didn't tell them that I felt abandoned all over again. They thought they were doing the thing that was in the best interest for me.

But I saw it differently.

I felt like I failed to be what they needed me to be so that they could love me. Again, there was something wrong with me.

After my aunt dropped me off at Boys Ranch in 1992, at the age of 12, I looked at the calendar and saw that it was May 13th.

My father had died May 9th, four years prior.

I started having an irrational fear of the month of May. I still do. Again, my life was completely changed a couple of weeks before my birthday. How did all these adults in my life not see what they were doing to me?

So, at the age of 12, a couple of weeks before my 13th birthday, my life was completely changed again.

Would the same things happen to me at this boys' home that happened to me at the last? I was bound and determined that they would not.

I would fight. Every day I would fight.

And I did. I fought everyone. It's all the control I had. And it helped get the anger out for a little while.

So, started my time at Cal Farley's Boys Ranch. A time that was to actually become a blessing, but which, on that mid-May day, I didn't see it as such.

Going to sleep that first night in my new home, I looked up at the ceiling and felt that old familiar feeling again. I was alone. All alone again.

Surrounded by other hurting boys, I was completely alone, and didn't belong anywhere, or with anyone.

My father was the last person in my life who wanted me, and he had been gone almost exactly four years.

Again, I was alone.

Chapter 7

Cal Farley's Boys Ranch is a real oasis in the northwest Texas Panhandle.

Situated in the Canadian River Valley, it was a young boy's paradise. The Ranch sat next to the slowly meandering red waters of the Canadian River. We would swim in those waters in the unbearably hot summers, trying to dodge the quicksand, and turned our skins red from the clay bottom that gave the river its distinctive color. Don't get me wrong, I felt such panicked loneliness at times during my stay at the Ranch, but it really was the best place for me. I would look back on my time there with a fondness that overshadows everything else in my younger life. I will say this over and over—it will always be my home. Whatever I can do for the Ranch in return for my time spent there, I will do with relish and happiness.

Large, old, venerable cottonwood trees would release their summer snow in the form of blowing cotton at the Ranch. By my birthday every year, I would know summer was in full swing when that blowing cotton would make it look like it had snowed all around us. There were so many tall healthy trees, the grass was amazingly green and deep and soft, and the smells of the surrounding country still linger in my memories to this day. All the buildings at the ranch were built with the same reddish Colorado River stone and made you realize that this place had a real heft, a real history. And it did. The beauty of the valley was only heightened by the constant winds that would blow across the Llano Estacado, or the plateau that made up most of the northern Texas panhandle.

Driving the very dangerous road from Amarillo to Boys Ranch, Texas Route 1061, also called Tascosa Road, you will see unbelievable sights.

An old, rich, oil-boom family from Amarillo bought land along the road going out to Boys Ranch and built things like "The Floating Mesa" and a deep valley with painted boulders, which resembled a giant pool table. The land was covered in cactus and scrub grasses. Mesquite trees, which were not native to the area, flourished. The story goes that mesquite beans would be caught up in the hooves of cattle being driven through the area up from Houston to the Kansas markets more than 100 years before my first trip out to the Ranch. The land was beautiful, and dangerous if caught out in it. Strong summer storms would sweep through, bringing hail, lightening, and sometimes tornados. All this wild beauty was so different from the concrete jungles I grew up in in North California. I was to learn the western way of life. I was to learn what being a man was all about, from men who came from the same areas of Texas that I was now a part of. I would come to take that history as my own. Later in life, when asked where I was from, I always answered, "Texas". The slow, easy, but hard-working life would become my legacy. I grew up on a real working ranch, and everything that went along with that.

In the 1930's, a local celebrity and business owner realized the needs of the sometimes parent-less boys running around Amarillo. He first sponsored an athletic club called Kid's Inc. I was a part of that club when I lived with my aunt and uncle. But it wasn't enough. He sent out word to his cohorts, and a man he knew named Julian Bivins donated an old ghost town site and the surrounding 120 acre of land he owned northwest of the city. It was the site of the old-west town called Tascosa. Many stories came from the time when that cattle town was

49

active. All that was left was the courthouse, the school, and a couple of other dilapidated buildings and many mesquite trees. They eventually had to build a bridge over the Canadian River to get out to the future site of Boys Ranch.

Cal Farley saw the place for what it could eventually become. A real home for as many wayward boys as he could find. And for the next 80 years, that's exactly what it became. The history of Boys Ranch is well known and can be found online and by visiting. Ranchers are available to this day to give visitors tours of the place, a job I had for many summers while I was there. The legacy of Cal Farley and the vision he had, as well as the ideals of Christian study, hard work, and lots of love and support for the boys are all still very apparent there. Many, many boys came to call the Ranch home, and I am one of them. I spent a little more than five years there, a very short part of my life, but the impact of the place will always allow me to answer the follow up question after "where in Texas?" as Cal Farley's Boys Ranch.

In recent times, there have been ex-ranchers coming out in the news describing abuse they suffered out at the Ranch. We all knew things like that were happening. Boys will always be the cruelest to each other. And through the years, there have been staff members who were not the best kinds of people. But everything I saw there shows me that for many boys, it was an amazing place, and a home, that taught us all how to work hard, and to accept the values that would make us successful as adults.

That's what I took from my experiences there, and while I have sympathy for the ones who faced abuse, I knew only support and willingness to teach me how to be a good man.

I took complete advantage of all the opportunities the Ranch provided, which a lot of boys did not. I eventually learned the benefits of the Ranch and kept with me many of the lessons I learned. They helped make me who I am today.

A huge part of being able to get through the traumas of early adulthood came from the strength I gained by being a Boys Rancher. If I can say anything about the Ranch, it would be a huge "Thank You".

I have not been vocal on the alumni pages online or spoke to the articles coming out about abuses experienced out at the Ranch by several boys, but I can honestly say that I gained much more than I lost by living there.

As a new kid who just arrived, with a chip on his shoulder, and anger enough for any three people, they really did the right thing with me.

They involved me in activities that would force me to learn responsibility and drive.

Within the first two weeks, they put me in a class called Horsemanship. I was taught for the first time in my life how to be around horses. I learned to ride, care for, and feed the large animals. I was frightened of them at first, but I learned something about myself in those weeks.

I loved animals. Absolutely loved them. Horses, dogs, calves. Caring for an animal will teach a young boy a lesson he really needs.

I also learned to be in control of something bigger than myself, a lesson that completely resonated with me. Controlling a large animal like a horse, making him go where you want him to go, and to go at the speed you tell him to go, will give a boy who has had no control over anything in his life an almost sense of being needed.

I would take different horses on a ride almost weekly for the next five summers. I rode bulls in two of the annual rodeos.

Of course, there were weeks of preparation and competition before you made it into the actual rodeo. I learned how to "green-break" untrained horses. I grew up in that country-like atmosphere that was so unlike anything else I knew.

I thought I was a tough kid from the city in California, but I learned what real strength was.

I became a cowboy. I didn't even know what a cowboy was, but I liked it. I could still listen to my kind of music, and like things like sports and cars, and technology, but deep inside, I learned pride, and have always considered myself a cowboy, if not in looks, then definitely in ideals and manners.

I also started to make friends. We were all kind of in the boat together. It sometimes felt like being in prison, or a concentration camp, because there were so many rules, and not much freedom.

I made friends that would stick with me for the rest of my life. One such friend was a girl by the name of Mary Vega. She was a staff girl, and was the most sarcastic, energy-driven girl I had ever met. She was a bit of a tomboy. She rode in the rodeo and played a couple of sports. She had a huge head of tight curly brown hair, and a cute little pixie face. She also had a big butt and loved to talk about how big it was.

I loved her like a sister, and she would see me in the hallways of the school and would always comment on me having my nose in a book.

I remember her asking me one time how many books I had read in my life. I couldn't give her a number and she just smiled at me and shook her head. Oh, if only she knew.

She was a special person, and she was the first girl I met in my life that I didn't want to kiss, but I loved her anyway. She was a beautiful girl. Sarcastic to a fault, and a little mean, but she had a heart everyone who knew her could see.

I didn't know it then, but she would be much more important in my life, many, many years down the road than I could ever have known.

There were many friendships forged by my time at the Ranch. I have so many brothers in my life that I don't know what to do with them all. And I would learn, as an adult, that we would all do absolutely anything for each other.

At Boys Ranch, I started to learn a thing about myself that had not been taught to me in the past, or if someone had tried to teach it to me, I was too caught up in the tragedy of my circumstances to recognize it.

That thing was pride.

I was encouraged to take part in team sports. I found out that I was good at softball and volleyball and was able to continue my love of swimming.

When I turned 13, I had to get a job, making a dollar an hour. I spent my first summer at the Ranch working with the horticulture crews.

I mowed lawns, trimmed trees, moved irrigation pipes, and cleaned out lakes. Taking care of the softball fields was a favorite job of mine. We would drag the infield, making it look perfect in preparation for the nightly intramural games between the many dormitories. I lived in MF dorm, and our colors were dark blue and white. We wore those colors with pride, and in my sophomore year, we won the softball championship, a huge feat. The picture of that team still sits in the trophy case of MF dorm the last time I visited.

During the next school year, 8th grade, I played basketball, and ran track. I also transitioned to a job working in the dining hall and found my love of cooking.

I found out something else about myself during this time. I could run. I could run for long periods of time, and I found great stamina within myself.

During this time, I was able to turn my anger into positive competition.

I wasn't the best at any one sport; there were more than 500 boys out there.

It was like having 500 older brothers.

But I was competitive and found pride in the sports I played.

I also hit puberty during 8th grade. I hit it hard. The summer between 8th grade and 9th grade I grew almost 6 inches.

My body lengthened out, I got taller, stronger, and more comfortable with myself. All of this helped me do better and better in sports. At the end of 8th grade, the annual intramural track meet was held. I ran in the 800m and the 1600m. I won both events and gained the attention of the varsity cross country coach.

He came up to me after the 1600m and told me that I needed to try out for the cross-country team at the end of the summer. Which I did, and I made the team.

I ran cross country for four years. I earned over 50 medals and ran all the way up to the Regional competition most of the years I ran. And one year we won the State Championship.

I also made the 9th grade basketball team, and tried out for tennis, a sport I had always loved watching. I made all of those teams, and my entire high school career was busy with sports.

I was also involved in non-athletic clubs. I was a four-year editor of the yearbook. I was on the speech and debate team, and in my senior year, a member of the one act play cast. During 8th and 9th grades I was in band. I played the alto saxophone and really enjoyed travelling with the band to football games. I had to drop it once I got involved in high school sports, but my love of music never went away.

My favorite part about being at Boys Ranch was the Chapel program. I was a part of everything from the choir, to the puppet ministry we had for one year. While I had grown up in church with my father, I was now learning about the love of God at Boys Ranch and learning that God is in control of all of this. They would talk about how we must surrender our lives to God and receive the Holy Spirit. I thought I had a relationship with Jesus Christ, but I would learn a very hard, valuable lesson towards the end of my 20's that would show me I didn't know Jesus like I thought I did.

It was this early immersion in Christianity that helped me eventually become the man of faith I am today.

Every Christmas, we held an annual cantata. I was a part of five of them.

Christmas was always the most special time of the year at Boys Ranch. They also made your birthday special, but we waited all year for Christmas. The anticipation leading up to it made us feel like the children we were. Those emotions were what, I felt like, normal kids had for Christmas. Christmas was also the only time of the year that we could go home, if we had a home to go to.

I went every year to my aunt and uncle's home. It was always a tense time, but it was also very enjoyable. For at least 9 days out of the year, I felt like I was back with my real family. And to my aunt and uncle's credit, they made it special for me while I was there. I would see Glen and Rebecca again, and my other cousins.

Birthdays were also very special out at Boys Ranch. The one that stands out the most is my 15th birthday.

When it is your birthday, they announce it at breakfast first thing in the morning. If you had your birthday during the school year, then your teachers would make it special, but as my birthday was in the summer, I didn't get the attention in school.

In the evening of your birthday, the bakery in the chow hall would make you a cake, and there would be ice cream as well.

At your dorm that night after dinner, there would be your birthday party. The Ranch would buy you a present that you got to pick out from catalogues a month or so before the big day. You picked three things, so it was a surprise what you were given.

They did the same thing for Christmas.

On your birthday, you could invite two of your best friends from other dorms to your party, and for at least one day at the Ranch, you weren't part of the 500 boys.

You were special.

That sounds like you aren't considered the rest of the year, which isn't true. I always felt cared for at the Ranch. I was blessed to have the same houseparent's from 8th grade to my senior year. While very heavy handed with discipline and rules, these house parents at least gave me a sense of continuity that I had not had since my father passed away.

What made my 15th birthday so special is that I found that I had some real friends. The guys in the bakery, who, after that first summer, I worked with in the chow hall, didn't make me one of the generic cakes they made everyone else.

Usually the cakes had white frosting, with different colors used to write just a happy birthday and your first name on the top of the flat cake.

My cake for my 15th birthday was a dark green color, shaded with black, and the cake artist, Adrian Diaz, used a set of air brushes to make it look like two clawed hands were coming out of the middle of the cake, followed by a pair of sinister colored eyes still within the cake.

It was amazingly artistic and made me so proud that they went against the standard just for me. To this day, Adrian runs a custom cake business. He has an amazing talent.

When we got to the dorm for my birthday party, our usual house parents were out of town, and the assistant house parents were also not available.

So, Coach Sparks, my cross-country coach, oversaw the dorm for the night. Finding out it was my birthday; he drove down to the concession stands by the football field and had some of the older boys help him load the coke machine into the back of his truck. It was unprecedented. We hardly ever got to enjoy soda, and to not only have an amazingly original cake for my birthday, we also had soda, and Coach Sparks was amazingly cool to let us unwind a little and have some fun.

That birthday stands out amongst them all for how special I felt. I really felt loved and popular and special. It was a real turning point for me, and I cherish the memory to this day. While others reading this might not think those were very big things, in my life, they were huge.

Many things during this time really resonate with me as an adult and has impacted parts of all my relationships to come. One in particular.

When I was 13 years old, my dorm decided to go into Amarillo for a movie night. We never did this, so it was a really big deal. The movie that we went to see was "Pure Country" starring George Strait. The movie was very entertaining, and it was an exceptional job done by the country music singer, but what really stands out is the final song of the movie.

At the end, George Strait's character is singing in a concert, and in particular, to his lady love. The song he sang was called "I Cross My Heart."

This song has stuck with me for the last 27 years. Every time I have been in a relationship, I've tried to make it "our" song. It hasn't worked once. The song describes exactly how I want my relationship to be. The words are simple, the melody easy and light, but the message of the words are so damn strong to me. I yearn for that kind of connection with a woman. A little foreshadowing.... I've never had it.

My time at Boys Ranch was a time of seeing the world for the first time in color. My experiences there were not shadowed by my emotions and hurts. For the first time in a very long time, I could, and often did, get outside of my head and notice the world around me.

The physical environment at the Ranch was exceptional. It was horrendously hot in the summers, with the west Texas winds making it feel like a variable oven.

It snowed in the winters and was bitterly cold.

We walked everywhere we went. It was almost a mile from my dorm to the chow hall, and we walked that walk three times a day. By the time I left, all the dorms were getting kitchens installed in them, and the boys ate some meals there.

I sound like an old man when I say, "In my time" but it is true. I was there before a lot of the niceties they have now were put into place. We walked and walked every day, and then is sports, we ran and ran. I sometimes wonder how many miles are on my legs from my time at the Ranch.

I also answered the questions in my mind about my sexuality. I now knew I liked girls, and I liked them a lot.

Starting in high school, I seemed to always have a girlfriend from out of town who would exchange letters with me on a weekly basis. I had two shoe boxes full of letters I received out at the Ranch.

To local girls, we were safe, because we were out there with a bunch of boys, and the girls would not be worried about us cheating. It was difficult though, as we could not date, or take them places. We could just write, maybe see them at an off-Ranch sporting event or invite them for the twice a year dances held at the Boys Center.

I kissed the first girl I had ever kissed out at SMP (Scripture Memorization Program) camp during the summer before 9th grade. Her name was Kelly, and I just remember it being sloppy and wet. She wore Sunflowers perfume, and for the next couple of years, it seemed all the girls I "dated" wore the same perfume.

To this day, smelling it makes my knees weak.

Those times were so influential, and I can recall so much. I have found that when a young boy sees things at this critical age, between 12 and 16, it can really stick with him, and change his viewpoint on things in his future.

Another example of this is the movie I saw that would dictate my "type" of woman I dated as an adult. The movie came out in 1990 and was called "Pump up the Volume" with Christian Slater and Samantha Mathis.

Samantha's character was named Nora, and for the next 25 years, every woman I was serious about looked just like Nora. My close friends and family would make fun of me incessantly because of this comparison. But I couldn't help it.

I fell in love with Nora, and cemented my taste from her, from that movie. Looking at pictures of Nora to this day makes me smile. Add in the

Sunflowers perfume, and I'm instantly transported to my early teens and the hormones and experiences from then.

The chapel program had a competition of sorts. We called it SMP, or scripture memorization program. You would memorize a chapter of biblical verses every week, and recite them on Saturday mornings, hoping to earn enough points to attend summer camp at Lone Tree Bible Camp in Capitan, New Mexico during the summer. It was one of the highlights of our year.

There are many hills and woods dotting the Ranch. One hill screams in my memories. The hill right behind my dorm on which stood the very recognizable water tower. The hill is covered in yucca plants and scrub grasses. There's cactus and mesquite bushes. Trees dot it, and steep, dirt tails meander all over, often leading to the top, as well as to other hideouts that boys had made and used to play games, like capture the Flag and Manhunt, for years.

I often would have to do work on this hill when I got into trouble. They called it being on "restriction."

I was on restriction a lot.

You didn't have any privileges when you were on restriction, and you had to work from sunup to sundown. One such instance was the time I had to carry two five-gallon buckets up to the top of the hill, fill them with dirt and rocks, and carry them back down, where I would dump them between my dorm and the next one. While it was a pointless drill, it nonetheless gave me time to think of what I had done wrong.

After being at the Ranch for a couple of years, I started going to the top of the hill behind my dorm and there was a spot next to the water tower where I would sit and look out over the valley to the rim of the next valley many miles to the south.

I would sit in this place, on top of this hill, for hours on the weekends, when we had the freest time. I started, for the first time, thinking about my future and what I wanted to do with it. I would daydream about jobs, and girls, and what I would do when I got out of Boys Ranch.

That makes it seem like I was in some way a prisoner there. And I was. But it wasn't a very bad prison. There really wasn't anywhere else where I would do as good. I knew that. I knew that the Ranch was home.

For the first time in my young life, I learned meditation, and the strife for inner peace. I was calm up on top of that hill.

That hill was the highest point in the Canadian River valley. I call it Water tower hill.

I sat at the very top, next to the tall, white water tower, proudly displaying the BR brand in deep blue. The days were mostly slow, and hot, and I could smell the heat dissipating off the buildings and the land down below.

As I sat there in the late afternoons, the shadows lengthening, the insects chirping, I would gaze at the same thing across the valley. The southern wall of the oval shaped valley was made up by a tall mesa and running directly up the middle of it was the road that led from Boys Ranch back to Amarillo.

Route 1061, the most dangerous road in Texas.

I would sit on top of that brush covered hill staring at that road. It was just a gray colored ribbon running up the side of the red dirt mesa, many miles in the distance.

But it represented my future.

I would gaze at that road and visualize my future, especially the day I would drive away from the Ranch and start my adult life.

I would come to learn a simple truth about teenage boys. We yearned to be men. We never visualized being a man for anything like making money, having sex, being bigger and stronger and being in charge.

No, the reason most teenage boys want to be men is because being a man means one thing. Freedom.

As a child, and then as a teenager, there are always adults telling you what to do, how to do it, and when to get it done. We, wrongly, compared being a grown man with the freedom to do whatever we wanted. It takes the experience of actually being a man to learn that there is no real freedom in this life, and in this world. We are ruled by our responsibilities and the consequences of our actions and decisions.

But that realization is far removed from a 16 or 17-year-old boy who dreams of the freedom of driving his own car up that far-away hill, tires crunching on that blacktop, with nothing in front of him but the plans he has set for himself, and the goals he strives to meet. I would stare at that road and plan out my entire adult life.

It didn't turn out anything like what I envisioned, but I nonetheless sat on that hilltop and watched the movie of my future take shape in my mind.

I became introspective on top of that hill. I started realizing that my thoughts were moving from juvenile ideals to concrete terms that would stabilize my core beliefs.

In short, I became a man on top of that hill.

All teenage boys have a place, or a time, or an event that turns them to look inside. To start realizing who they are. When that happens, I think that that is when they truly can be called a man.

I also learned a thirst within me to make up stories. I started writing these stories down, and of course, I was continuing to read at a voracious rate.

There were so many books in the library at the high school, and I went through just about all of them.

During this time, my brother got me interested in fantasy novels. I started with Terry Brooks. Which led to Anne McCaffery and Robert Jordan. I reread Tolkien and got into comic books. I loved Superman. This would prove important later in life. But I started really letting my imagination run away with all these worlds of make believe. I started noticing that writers had voices. They wrote with personality, and I started learning the syntax and tools used to tell a proper story. My mind opened to the fact that maybe, just maybe, I was a storyteller myself. Careers were often spoken about, and when I said I wanted to be a writer, I was always encouraged to have something to fall back on. Which is a completely normal reaction to a child saying they want to be a writer when they grow up. It doesn't work for them all. Some just don't have the gift. At the same time, though, I had a couple of very influential English teachers who encouraged me to pursue my passion, even if it was only ever a hobby.

One professor, later in life in college, gave me the first and only real advice I would use to continue to write. I had written a 19k word short story and I asked Dr. Smith to read it. It was a rough draft, and I knew it wasn't the greatest thing I had ever written. But I was proud of it, and proud that I had written it in just a couple of evenings.

Dr. Smith, the Professor Emeritus of the English Department, sent me an email to talk about my short story. I nervously stepped into his office, ready to hear biting truth that I wasn't a talented enough writer. He handed me back my manuscript, and looking at the top page, there wasn't a red mark on it. I was confused. Surely, he would make all kinds of corrections. He told me to turn to

63

the last page for his synopsis. Under the last sentence of the story, in bold red pen, he wrote one line of review:

"Keep writing as much as you can! You have the gift…" Signed, Dr. Smith.

I couldn't keep the tears from my eyes and thanked him hurriedly. Walking down the hallway in that century-old building at the center of the campus of my school, I soared higher than I had ever soared before. I had a gift! And for the first time in my life, a purpose. Two weeks later, I started writing for the school's weekly newspaper. I had never had a paid writing gig before, but it showed me that one day, this is what I was made to do. All the way back at Boys Ranch, many years in the past, when I realized that I had stories in my mind to share, the connections from that long-ago day to the present one exposed what I needed to do with my life. Everything I am is dependent on that fact. I am a writer.

Sitting back on top of my hill, I would look out over the tapestry of the external world of Boys Ranch. That world is indelibly scorched onto my memories.

The warm air, the amazingly clean smells of the countryside, and the sights and sounds of the Ranch make me miss it to this day. There were once fruit trees in an orchard there. It was later built over for a middle school, but while all the trees were there, I learned the beauty of picking ripe fruit straight from the tree and enjoying it on the spot.

There were several apple trees scattered throughout the Ranch. These small, tart apples were original to Boys Ranch. I have never experienced them anywhere else in my life.

We would run by the trees during cross country practice and pick several apples apiece and eat them while we ran.

We would fish the ponds and lakes of the area during the summers. In the evenings was rodeo practice. Those of us riding the bulls and broncs would meet behind the chutes and prepare for one ride a night, in which we would be scored, and only the top twenty riders would get to participate in the actual Rodeo.

I rode in two of them before an accident when I was 16 stopped my rodeo career for life. I had drawn a twisted horn brahma bull named "Freckles."

Some of the older boys warned me that he would try to twist his head and hook one of my legs. Which is exactly what he did. He was an extremely strong bull, and while I stayed on as long as I could, he succeeded in hooking my left leg, pulling me off and under him, and proceeded to step on my left thigh, and my lower back.

I was taken straight to the clinic, and the next morning, when I urinated blood, I was taken to the hospital in Amarillo.

"Freckles" had created a massively swollen hematoma on my left thigh, which was beautifully bruised and stayed that way for a couple of weeks.

But my lower back, he did a real number on. Not only did he pop a hole in my left kidney, which fortunately clotted up and eventually healed, but he tore several of my lower back muscles, and to this day I still get frighteningly bad lower back pain.

Another big influence in my life during these years at the ranch was music. We were inundated with Christian music, which I loved, but I was also able to let my tastes move from classic rock, like White Snake and Aerosmith, to new age grunge like Nirvana. I loved country music and listened to Kenny Rogers and George Strait. I loved heavy metal bands like Ramstein and Type O Negative. I listened to Tom Petty and The Eagles pretty religiously. I bought CD's of Deep Blue Something, Live, and Boys to Men, Roxette, ABBA, and Counting Crows.

I tried a little bit of everything. I rocked out to Thugs Bones and Harmony, Coolio, and Snoop Dogg.

I really loved just about anything that made me happy, and music had a way to really make me happy. My tastes are very eclectic. I still listen to just about every kind of music.

I gravitate more towards 90's and early 00's music, but I will jam out to anything from the 50's to now. Playing in my earphones right now is Disturbed, followed by Pink, and then a song by Neil Diamond. A little bit of everything. I'm not ashamed that I don't home in on any one genre. I love music, period.

There were more than five years of memories at Boys Ranch. A lot of them were focused around hard work. When you have a teenage boy, who came from such brokenness, and had so much anger and animosity built up within him, the best thing to do is to keep him so busy and so tired that he doesn't think about his hurts.

It may not always work and doesn't get to the heart of the matter. It doesn't fix the hurt, but it does a good job of making him not wallow in his pains. For a lot of the time at the Ranch, I didn't feel those early feelings of loneliness.

I had made a lot of friends, and of course, after I had been there for about three months, my brother Jasper showed up.

His experiences at the Ranch were a lot different than mine. To him, the Ranch was a prison, and a daily torture.

Our relationship through the next four years would go back and forth between being as close as brothers could be, to being very strained as I tried to find my identity on my own.

Jasper's experiences would hinder a lot of the growth I was yearning to find. The men we both became would start right there, in that West Texas country.

And for all of us ex-ranchers, we either came out ahead, or stayed broken and bitter, using the experiences there to further our pains and frustrations.

It was a matter of degree. For some, it was home, and will always be.

For others, it was hell. And always would be.

Chapter 8

Before Jasper came to Boys Ranch, he had lived with my aunt and uncle, Travis, and Jenny. Travis was the opposite of the men I had lived around in Texas. He was studious, a bit nerdy, and very introverted. Jasper, by proxy, became much the same way. Travis never wrestled with Jasper. There wasn't any kind of kind-hearted bantering that showed he cared about the boy.

My uncle Jerold and his sons were very banal with me and let me be a little rough. To be a boy.

Jasper was isolated and given things like books and Legos. While I was crashing my bike and throwing papers for money, Jasper was in the house all the time, not learning social cues, and becoming introverted as well. I feel that the way Travis was as an example for Jasper made his life out at Boys Ranch very difficult. By the time he got to the Ranch, he was a complete nerd type. He just never belonged, and never made many friends.

Jasper was very co-dependent on me in those years we spent together at the Ranch. He didn't have any friends and was bullied constantly. I stood up for him as much as I could, but I was cruel to him too. We would argue terribly. At my semi-annual progress meetings, we had with my houseparent's and my aunt, and some of the supervision at the Ranch, it was often brought up how much Jasper depended on me for his identity and I was the only person he spent time with. He was often isolated and did things alone. He read even more than I did. I know he didn't go through the things I had gone through, but he went through a lot himself. He was never given an outlet for his feelings, and every time he showed anger, and acted out, they would just put him on restriction. They did the same thing to me, but for some reason, when I look back on those years, it was always harder on Jasper.

I pitied him, and really cared about him, but I was trying to find my own social identity and to grow up to be a good man. Jasper was often stuck in his own thoughts and demons. The older boys in the dorm picked on him mercilessly. He was mentored by one older boy, but when that boy graduated, Jasper was left on his own again.

I felt so sorry for him, and anger in how he was treated. But I was often unkind to him as well. Today, we are the best of friends, and have supported each other through all kinds of difficulties, but in those impressionable years, he had it unfairly difficult.

To put it into a proper picture, years later I would watch the movie, "Napoleon Dynamite" and I saw my brother as he was in high school. It was a perfect portrayal of him, even his mannerisms.

Jasper went on to have a very distinguished career as a combat medic in the United States Navy. He grew into an amazing man. He has a penchant for women and used to live a lifestyle I don't always agree with, but he is incredibly generous and loving. He obviously overcompensated for his extremely heartbreaking experiences as a teenager, but he grew from them as well.

He also learned that he had inherent skills in dancing, lifting weights, and hair loss. He is a humongous, bald man now at the age of 41.

He is incredibly educated in the fields of medicine and industrial safety. He has three sons, and a very successful career, in which he is one of the youngest at his level.

69

He, more than anyone I have ever known, grew from his horrible experiences, and used them to strengthen his character, rather than let them get him down.

He rarely drinks, doesn't smoke, and has never done drugs. He is disciplined and lives by his own set of deep-seeded rules. He has never been in jail, or much trouble for that matter. He daily exceeds the statistics that says he should be having a bad adult life, considering his childhood.

He has been a stabling influence in my life, and I love him deeply. We have been there for each other through every bad thing, and I rely on him tremendously. After everything he's been though, he just radiates strength.

I do wish he were still a Christian, but he chose a different path years ago. We often argue about Jesus, and my faith-driven life choices, but he is still very supportive.

All I can say is that, yes, he had a miserable time at Boys Ranch, but he, too, used the experiences to drive him to succeed. I can say that him, more than anyone else in my life, pushes me to be better. I am so proud of him, and who he is.

My brother, just like me, is a fighter. He learned that.

My father had been a military man, and Jasper and I both did our duty in the service.

One situation at Boys Ranch sticks out in my memory. Jasper and I were in the same room in MF dorm for a time. The other boy in the room was named Eric. Eric was a cowboy and was extremely good at both bull riding and bronc riding. He was tall, and older than us, and was not a nice person at all.

One night, when my brother had gotten out of the shower, Eric started popping him with a towel. Flicking it against Jasper, it was drawing welts on his back, and he was close to crying. I was sitting on my bed holding my tennis racket, and when Eric looked over at me, he asked me if I wanted to hit him. I said I did. But I didn't have the guts to. Eric was a dangerous person. He picked on Jasper relentlessly.

This went on for a couple of years. Jasper never got revenge, but always spoke about what he would do to Eric if he could.

Eric got taken out of Boys Ranch a little later, and the summer after I graduated, I got a call in my dorm room in college from my old houseparent.

She informed me that Eric had been killed in a motorcycle accident.

I, deep in my heart, was almost glad about it. I felt shame for feeling those feelings, but I had them. I called Jasper, who was stationed in California at the time, and told him the news.

Uncharacteristically, or at least as I saw it should be, Jasper was quiet. I asked him if he was secretly glad like I was, and all he said was,

"No, I'm not glad. I hope his family is okay. And I hope Eric is at peace now."

I was floored. If anyone should be happy about the death of Eric, it was my brother. But my brother showed compassion and maturity far beyond his age.

I learned a lot about my brother Jasper in that moment. I learned that he overcame his experiences at the Ranch and was a much better man than me. He wasn't a Godly man, but he was a man full of compassion and grace, and forgiveness. That was a lesson it would take me many more years to master. But my brother did it, against all odds. That is the man my brother turned into.

I don't want to get into the many more instances of bullying my brother faced. I know I wasn't always kind to him, and often chided him during high school to try to be cooler. To try to not be such a dork. To not have the reputation he did.

I didn't know, at the time, how to accept him for who he was, or to see who he was becoming. I just felt like he was dragging me down.

I wasn't the most popular person at the Ranch, but I wasn't in the social hell my brother was in. I was an athlete, and high up in my class rankings, academically wise.

My brother didn't blossom until he left the Ranch and joined the military.

He found himself in the fields of Japan and South Korea, where he would train alongside the Marine platoons he oversaw, medically.

And he became a hero in Iraq, when he saved many lives during a roadside bombing against the convoy he was riding in.

He was decorated, and a book should be written about his life.

Many heroes were made in the desert of Iraq, but none of them are my big brother.

Jasper Fox will always be a hero in my book.

Napoleon Dynamite became a badass!

Chapter 9

My brother was at Boys Ranch with me for four years. He graduated in 1996 and within a year, joined the Navy.

I prepared for my senior year. I was secretly excited to be there without my brother, but I soon missed him very much.

My senior year was a whirlwind of activities, and it culminated of course with my graduation.

I can give one example of the differences between the times I had at the Ranch compared to my brother's. At his graduation, only one family member came to see him walk across the stage. I was there, of course, but my uncle Travis was the sole member of our family that came to wish Jasper well.

He drove Jasper into Amarillo and dropped him at the apartment my brother had set up to live in with a roommate. That was it.

At my graduation, I had my aunt and uncle, Glen and Rebecca, my best friend, Ruth, five members of the Staff family, and my brother came back from the Navy to see me walk the stage.

I'm not explaining the differences here to gloat, rather to show the stark differences in his experience there compared to mine. I will take some time here to explain who the Staff family was, as well as my best friend Ruth.

My brother had to have reconstructive surgery to his left knee during his junior year in high school. While he was being taken into Amarillo twice a week for physical therapy, he met a girl named Mia Staff. Mia was a gregarious girl a year younger than Jasper, but they hit it off, and Jasper had his first girlfriend. They got on well, and her family kind of adopted Jasper, and eventually, me. Even after Jasper broke Mia's heart, the Staff family were very kind to me. I connected well with Mia's mother, Kris. We spoke for hours at a time, and I learned a lot from her.

The father, Craig, was an engineer, and was wicked smart. I also got along well with him. They had three children in all, and Mia's little brother and sister were equally awesome to me.

In fact, the summer after graduation, the Staff family allowed me to live with them until I started college in the fall. My aunt and uncle met the Staff's and they all liked each other. I was very blessed to know the Staff's, and I still am. While tragedy and blessings follow just about every family, the Staffs have had their dose of both through the years. I'm not as close to them as I once was. Mia still calls me brother when I speak to her, and Kris is still just as full of life as she always was.

During a football game one Friday night at Boys Ranch, I noticed a beautiful girl I had never seen before sitting in the stands. She was sitting on the home team side, so she had some affiliation with Boys Ranch.

The night was clear. The stars shown bright, and we won the game against nearby Spearman. It was a great night, and for some reason the universe aligned just right to give me the opportunity to speak to this beautiful girl I couldn't take my eyes from.

While I was walking back to my dorm after the game, I noticed the girl walking towards the dorms up a different street. I quickly caught up with her. It was a weird enough sight to see a girl walking alone at Boys Ranch, let alone one who didn't belong there.

I asked her if she was ok and needed any help. She told me she was walking up to a dorm to visit with her friend, Olin Reynolds. I knew Olin, didn't really care much for him, and was intrigued how this wonderful girl knew him.

To this day I don't remember what she told me, but I told her I would walk her to the dorm, and make sure she made it safe. It gets very dark in areas of Boys Ranch, so I knew she would be walking through some areas that while safe, would still require some care.

We didn't have long to talk, so I let her ask me who I was, where I was from, and what I liked about the Ranch. I, of course, asked her how she found herself there that night, and I found out that she was the daughter of a distinguished alumni.

That made sense. Why else would she know anything about the Ranch?

I found talking to her to be extremely comfortable, and her presence, and warmth of spirit just radiated from her. And did I mention how beautiful she was?

She told me her name was Ruth Scott, and I will admit, I was smitten then and there. As we walked up to Olin's dorm, I drew up the courage to ask for her phone number. She gave it, and I jotted it down on the paperback book I was carrying, which was just one in a long line of books I always had with me.

I vowed to call her the next day, as it was a weekend, and we could use the phone for 15 minutes. I dropped her at the door of the dorm, and she gave me a hug. She smelled amazing, and I marveled that this creature existed.

The next day I called her, of course, and what followed for the next two years was just the most amazing friendship I've ever had. Ruth was such an amazing girl.

While she made it clear from the very beginning that we would not be dating, I still couldn't help falling in love with her. She was an amazingly strong Christian, as well as had the kindest soul I have ever encountered.

I learned that her mother had married the Boys Ranch Alumni, and he wasn't Ruth's biological father. She had a younger sister and brother. Her brother had autism, and the times I would visit Ruth at her home in Amarillo, he and I got along very well.

Ruth's family lived within a mile of the Staff's in Amarillo, so the summer after high school, I spent equal time between the two houses.

Ruth's mother, Cyndi, and her adopted father owned a windshield repair company. The only two employees were Ruth's parents. Until that summer. They hired me at the start of the summer, and I worked with them until I left for college.

It was the best summer of my life. I saw Ruth every day and made good money while learning a new trade.

They welcomed me as a son. I think there was a lot of pressure for Ruth and me to end up together, but I always felt that she was too good for me. I professed to be a Christian, but I knew in my heart that I had not given my life to Christ. I was too selfish.

I was still a virgin, but that was more by a lack of opportunity than actual spirituality. I would get a couple of opportunities to lose my virginity around the time I started college, but to me, there really wasn't a rush. I claimed to be a Christian, but I didn't fully believe it on the inside. I had even been baptized when I lived with my aunt and uncle, but it wasn't real. That would come in my late 20's, and that is an amazing story, soon to come.

One experience stands out from that summer. Ruth's dad and I had often talked about how I could get Ruth to date me. I wanted her to see me as a possible boyfriend, rather than just her best friend. And we were best friends. We spent all our time together and talked so much.

I told her a lot of what had happened to me as a child, which I had never done with anyone else before, and she told me a lot about her own struggles and experiences growing up.

She was incredibly kind and was just a very special person. I could see that from the first time we met.

Her birthday was approaching that summer, and it just happened to coincide with Garth Brooks being in concert in Amarillo. He was there, playing at the baseball stadium in downtown Amarillo for two nights. The second night happened to be her birthday. Her father and I put together a plan.

He would give me my paycheck early so that I could surprise her with tickets to the concert on her birthday. But we told her that we were unable to get the tickets. I told her I had a plan though. She loved Garth Brooks, and just wanted to hear him. Right behind the baseball stadium, was the Coke a Cola bottling plant. I had a friend that worked there, and several of the employees were bringing their families and setting up chairs in the parking lot of the plant. While we couldn't see what was going on in the concert, we could hear it quite well. I planned for her and me to set up some lawn chairs next to my car in this parking lot, and she seemed quite pleased with the experience.

We listened to the first night's concert there in that parking lot, and Ruth, being the kind girl she was, told me that it was a great birthday present that I would set that up for her. I had some snacks with us, and we had a bit of a picnic. What she didn't know, is that I spent my entire two weeks' pay on up-front tickets to the next night's show, in the VIP section.

The next day, her father let me borrow a Garth Brooks t-shirt he had, and I wore my boots and cowboy hat. I told her I was taking her out for a birthday dinner, and her parents pretended that they had some important things come up that night and that she should go with me, and they would make it up to her later.

77

I pulled up to her house in my little red car and rang the doorbell in my tight wrangler jeans, boots, cowboy hat, and country music t-shirt. She had never seen me decked out in cowboy clothes, and I must say, I cut a dashing figure. But Ruth. Man did she clean up well. She was wearing her favorite purple country top, and tight blue jeans. I told her we were going country dancing. Something I really enjoyed doing every Sunday night, and she didn't question the clothing choices.

I pulled up to the baseball stadium, and the tickets I had purchased gave us choice parking. She was surprised, and when I told her that I had, in fact, gotten tickets, she was very pleased. And when I led her to the seats, I was so proud of the shock she showed. She held my hand and was very affectionate throughout the concert. Garth Brooks gave an amazing performance, as he always did in those years, and it was just a magical night. It was a night I would think back on many times in the years to come.

One circumstance stands out from that night the most. There was an older man sitting behind our seats, and during one of the breaks in the music, he tapped us both on the shoulder. He had a rather large camera, and he asked if he could take our picture. We agreed, and after taking several shots, he told us that we were just the most beautiful couple he had seen. And as I looked over at Ruth, I didn't correct the man. We were a beautiful, young couple. We weren't together, but our bond and connection could be seen by those who knew what to look for. Within a month, I would lose Ruth forever, by my own choices, and it was the worst mistake I ever made.

And so, we go back to the afternoon of my high school graduation. I was surrounded with support and love.

After saying my goodbyes of everybody I had come to love in my time there, I climbed into my over-packed little red Ford Aspire hatchback and drove away from my home.

At the southern end of the valley, as my car tires crunched on the hard blacktop and I climbed that hill out of view of the Ranch, I felt the hairs on the back of my neck stand up, and I could see the thick, invisible line of memory, stretching from me, on that day, to the young man sitting on top of the hill behind me for so many hot afternoons, and it all came home.

Two tears fell from my eyes, and my throat tightened up. But I smiled.

Mentally letting go of that boy on top of that hill and turning at the top of the red dirt mesa, I gladly drove my little car quickly into my future.

I did not look back.

Chapter 10

In the fall, I would be moving into the college dorms at West Texas A&M University, in Canyon, Texas, about 15 miles south of Amarillo. It was close by, and I was extremely excited to start.

Ruth was a year behind me in school, so she would be starting her senior year at her high school in Amarillo. I planned to still see her every chance I got, but I knew with classes starting up, and keeping up my grades so that I maintained my scholarships was going to be a lot of work. I wanted to start college a way I had never started anywhere before. I wanted to stand out, socially, and let the confidence I had found during my senior year, and the following summer, to bolster my status at the small West Texas A & M University.

I had enrolled as a Pre-law major. I was following the advice of several of my teachers from the Ranch, as well as my houseparent's and other staff who all felt that I would make an amazing lawyer. I had already been in touch with Texas Tech's School of Law in Lubbock, and that was the destination goal after my first four years in college.

I had it all planned out and was ready to start on the journey. When I left for college in late August, I had the whole world in front of me. I was single, in great shape, looking forward to the academic challenges ahead. I had graduated in the top 10% of my class, and I knew that I had the tools to be as successful as I wanted to be. Ruth supported me in my career choice and had even talked at great lengths about how I could be a Christian lawyer, and really work for the underdogs who needed me. I was idealistic, and on a mission. It all started with the day I moved into Gunther Dorm on the campus of WTAMU. Almost from the first day, I became such an outgoing and outrageously friendly freshman.

During the first week leading up to classes starting, the college held a freshman orientation week. It was called Buff Branding. The mascot at WT was the buffalo. There were lots of group games, as well as information about going to college. Every evening there was a concert on the green, or a dance, and one night was a massive party, just for the entering freshman class.

At the end of the week, they held an awards ceremony, and gave out the ultimate award, the distinguished Buff Brander. One went to a male freshman, the other went to a female. I, of course, won the men's prize for having the most school spirit. I entered school with a couple of other guys from Boys Ranch, who I had grown up with. At the Ranch, they were more popular than me, but at WT, I started my reputation the right way. I was so outgoing, many of the freshman girls did not want to approach me. I could see the social standings lining up the same way they did in high school.

During that first week, we were told to go to the main administration building to sign up for our classes that semester. I stood in line with all the other students, waiting my turn at the computers to sign up for classes. This was before the times when all students had laptops, and access to the internet. This was before smart phones, and wireless internet. At WT, I had my first email address. I had never sent an email before 1997.

While standing in line, I felt a tap on my shoulder. I turned around and there was Tonya. We had met during the summer. We were both entering freshmen and were the only two Pre-law majors. We spent a day together meeting professors during one of the several orientations before starting the school year.

I said hello, and she introduced me to the girl standing next to her. The girl was her little sister, and I found out her name was Victoria.

She was a mousy little thing. She was wearing a pair of jean overalls over a dark blue shirt, and the cuffs at the bottom were rolled up, showing white deck shoes and low-rise white socks. She was very pretty in a waspish way and had gorgeous eyes.

She looked nothing like her sister, Tonya, but I knew what that was like, as my brother and I look nothing alike.

I got to the computer, and accidently bumped into Victoria. I think I made her mad and didn't really think anything of it afterwards. I signed up for my classes, got my printout, and saying goodbye, I turned and left. She was out of my mind before I even walked back out into the hot Texas sunshine.

Two nights later, there was a concert on the green. It was a local Christian rock band, and the music was loud, and everyone was excited and happy, and jumping around to the beat. I was in my element. By this time, all the freshmen knew me, and I was getting high-fives and talking to as many people as I recognized. I made my way to the front of the sizable crowd of students, and as I looked up at the band on the makeshift stage set up between two dorms, I was having the time of my life.

Eventually I looked around me, as it got darker, and the lights of the Green came on. There were stage lights as well, sweeping the crowd of students, and making it seem like a real concert, there in the middle of the college campus.

At the edge of the Green was a row of trees, and I made my way over to their shade. Someone had set up some large orange jugs of what appeared to be lemonade, and I was thirsty.

I got my plastic cup of the sweet drink, and I looked up and saw the same mousy girl leaning up against one of the trees near the drink tables.

It was Victoria, and she was visibly upset. Tears were streaking down her face, and I felt something tearing at my heart at seeing her in pain. I didn't know her, but something drew me to her.

I approached her and bent down to yell in her ear over the music. I asked her if she was ok, and she just shook her head. The music was obviously Christian, and I thought maybe she was having a spiritual movement. She just kept crying and shaking her head. There was no way I could hear her over the loud music, so I put down my cup, took her by the hand, and pulled her after me to somewhere quiet.

To this day, I have no idea why I did those things. Looking back, after everything I know now, I could see fate's hand on us that night.

I had several people who knew me at this point. I had the Staff family in Amarillo to support me, as well as Ruth, and her parents. There were many staff members at the Ranch rooting for my success, and my own family was still in the picture, in some small ways. For the first time in my life, I was surrounded by concerned people, who wanted the best for me. I had so much support.

At that time, I wasn't even thinking about the childhood I had had to endure. My father's death was years behind me, and I had worked hard to have people in my life who loved me and wanted the best for me.

But I didn't think of any one of those people that night.

If I had just thought of any one of them, and what they would think about what I would do over the next 6 months, I wouldn't have taken Victoria by the hand.

I wouldn't have talked to her late into that night.

I wouldn't have walked around campus with her until the sun came up the next day.

I wouldn't have kissed her on the steps of the museum.

If I would have thought of Ruth's opinion in that moment, I wouldn't have even put my lemonade down and tried to find out what was bothering this girl.

If I knew what was in store for me over the next eight years with this girl, I wouldn't have cared why she was crying, and better yet, I would have run as far away as I could.

If I knew what would happen between Ruth and me because of this girl, I would have gone straight to Amarillo that night and begged Ruth to forgive me.

My life was irrevocably changed that late summer night.

My carefully planned out future would never be realized, and it all started that warm, sweet night, under the trees on the campus of WTAMU, and I would forever be changed by it.

I didn't know it at the time, but I would lose everyone.

Chapter 11

Over the next several weeks, Victoria and I became severely co-dependent on each other. We spent every waking moment together that we weren't in class. We spoke on the phone when we weren't physically in each other's presence, and we did all this to the exclusion of everyone we knew.

I had rushed a fraternity, Kappa Sigma, and she became a Kappa sweetheart. As the days turned colder outside, and the trees started losing their leaves, we fell in what we thought was love with each other. I started hearing whisperings from my friends and frat brothers that Victoria had a little bit of a reputation there in town.

Apparently, she had quite a few trysts with guys from another frat before she met me and had also been with a couple of guys that worked out in Palo Duro Canyon, at an outside theatrical show called "Texas", where she had worked the previous summer.

I ignored all these warnings from my friends. Here was a girl who was showing me attention and wanted the same things in life that I thought I did. Namely, a family, and to be more adult then we were at the time.

We made several bad decisions and broke the rules about girls staying in the guy's dorm rooms. For the first time in my life, I was sexually intimate with a girl, although it was still important to me that I remain a virgin.

We did everything else imaginable together though. I felt like I wanted to marry her, and I knew that she wanted to marry me.

We were on cloud 9 getting the attention from each other that we had always needed. I was so excited about being with her.

I told my friends and family. They were all very hesitant and reminded me to focus on my classes. I had a goal in mind, a life planned out, and I was allowing this girl to come in and start interrupting the plan. I didn't care. Someone loved me, and was attracted to me, and I threw caution to the wind.

I was, however, involved in quite a few clubs that semester.

Greeks for God, Kappa Sigma, I was elected president of my dormitory. I was on the student round table as well as another prayer group that met twice a week.

I took Victoria to all these events and gatherings, but I knew that I was burning myself out.

Classes were rough, because no one was making me go to them, and I often skipped. I just wanted to spend all my time with this girl. She felt the same way, and we were very immature and unhealthy in the amount of time we spent together.

She was a part of a Church of Christ student group, and we went away with them to New Mexico to a couple's retreat in the mountains for a weekend.

There were a lot of biblical based lectures on how to have a Godly relationship, and we took part in a couple of strengthening exercises for couples.

One excercise stands out in my memories, and again, it showed that we should have not headed down the road we went down.

In this exercise, one large tree was at the end of a clearing. About 40 yards from it, stood two other trees, about 30 feet from each other. There were two heavy wires anchored into the lone tree, about three feet off the ground. The two wires were anchored into the tree right next to each other, and extended outwards towards the other two trees, making a triangle between the three trees.

The object was for a couple to stand on the wires at the lone tree, and holding each other up, start slowly scooting along the wires, moving further and further apart. You had to rely on your partner to hold you up as you moved further away from each other. The lesson with this exercise was to see if you could trust your partner to hold up your weight as you had to extend further and further out from each other.

Every couple there did not make it very far in this exercise. Victoria and I made it about halfway between the trees, but we failed because I didn't trust her strength to hold up my weight, and she didn't trust me to keep her steady. The couple who made it almost the whole way, extending almost parallel to the ground, was me and another guy about my size. We did it for fun, but it was interesting to see that we made it further than anyone else. I knew he was strong enough to hold up my weight, and vice versa. It was an object lesson that stayed with me for a long time. It was all about trusting your partner and believing in their strength.

We had a photo of Victoria and me on those wires, talking to each other as we moved farther apart. The look on her face as I stood in front of her was frustration and a little bit of determination. My body language showed that I was trying to do all the work of balancing and holding us both up.

Those feelings would dominate our next eight years together. Her being frustrated at me, and me trying to hold everything together. It was a mixture doomed to fail. I just wasn't responsible or mature enough to see it back then.

Towards the middle of that first semester, as Victoria's birthday came closer, and I became more and more uninterested in college, I received a phone call from Ruth.

Our friendship had become strained since Victoria and I started seeing each other. I didn't give Ruth all the details and didn't tell her about the sexual stuff that Victoria and I had been doing. I felt that Ruth would have judged me very harshly for that.

During the phone call, Ruth asked me if I could come to Amarillo the next evening and drive her to the airport. She was flying to see her biological father and wanted me to drive her. I assumed she needed some support for the trip and wanted to talk to her best friend about it. I was very wrong.

As we drove towards the Amarillo Airport, Ruth was quiet. I could tell something was on her mind, but I didn't pry. That wasn't the way between us. Eventually, she reached into her purse and pulled out a plain white envelope. It was sealed and had my name on the front of it. She placed it between us and told me to read it after I left her at the gate. I proceeded to tell her that that was not the way it was between us, and since we were a little early for her flight, I pulled into a parking lot right off I-40. I put the car in park and looked over at her. I asked her to read me the letter.

She was hesitant at first, but knew that our relationship, and how much we trusted each other and told each other everything, dictated that it was safe and ok to read me what was inside the envelope. She tore open the envelope, pulled out a nicely folded letter, written in her beautiful handwriting, and started to read.

The letter she wrote me started out by telling me how much she valued me in her life. I was touched and interrupted her to tell her I felt the same way about her. She was my best friend, and always would be. She shushed me and asked if I could not say anything until she finished reading me the letter. I agreed and was quiet until she finished. I was even quieter after she was done.

The letter went on to tell me exactly how she really felt. She said in the letter that she had been in love with me since we met. She loved me deeply, and I was everything to her. And now she felt like she had lost me because of my relationship with Victoria and asked me if I could end things with Victoria to be with her. She described how she knew I loved her as well, always had, and she just took it for granted that we would end up together, because that's what she prayed for every night, and had been cautious about telling me how she really felt because of her faith. She knew we belonged together, and we would support each other through school, and careers, and we would have a beautiful family one day together.

I was stunned. Too stunned to speak. I knew that if I left Victoria and started a romantic relationship with Ruth, it would be slow, methodical, and wouldn't have the physical aspect that I had with Victoria. Ruth just wasn't like that. She was pure, and innocent, and knew one day those things would be important, but for now, her faith and relationship with Christ would preclude any kind of physicality between us. But she was the girl of my dreams, everything I had ever wanted in a soulmate, and I was going to get back to Canyon and break things off with Victoria immediately. I asked Ruth if we could talk when she got back the next week. I told her I would pick her up when she flew back into Amarillo and tell her what I wanted to do at that time.

I dropped her off at the airport in a daze. I sat in my car and reread the letter twice. I felt a burning in my chest reading her beautiful words. I realized this was exactly what I wanted to hear from Ruth for two solid years. I thought back to my graduation day, when she had worn a tight, amazing red dress, and turned every head around her. She exuded a calm and beauty that was entirely too good for me. I still knew in my heart that I wasn't good enough for her, but she saw me differently. She saw the real me. No one else would see me like that until I was 40 years old, and a world and lifetime away from that night, in my car, confused about what I should do. Her maturity and faith were evident in the letter. She had a mature understanding of where her life was heading, and she wanted me in it. At that moment, I should have done something I wasn't very good at. I should have prayed for guidance. I should have asked God what decision I should make. But I didn't. To my detriment, I did not ask God for any help.

I drove back to Canyon, and when I got to my dorm room, I called Victoria. I told her we needed to talk. I asked her if she would like to go for a drive. She agreed, and I drove to her dorm and picked her up. When she got in the car, she commented on how she could smell Ruth's perfume still lingering. She sounded jealous, and I knew she didn't like my relationship with Ruth. I drove away, in my thoughts, and not saying anything to her for a few minutes.

She asked me what was wrong, and I handed her the beautiful letter that my best friend had written, just for me. Victoria read it, and I glanced over at her as she went from one page to the next. I saw tears forming in her eyes, and one fell onto the pages in her hand.

She finished the letter and looked over at me with red, tear streaked eyes, and her makeup running down her cheeks. I pulled over into the Walmart parking lot, more miles away from the campus then I realized. I parked under the lights and killed the engine. It was cool enough outside that just cracking the windows made it comfortable inside my little car.

She asked me what I was going to do. I didn't know how to respond. I knew in that moment that she was aware of how I felt about Ruth. She could tell from the things I told her about our relationship together. She had met Ruth, and the friction between the two of them was palatable. Victoria at that moment did the only thing she knew how to do. She reached over the space between us and started kissing me.

My body responded, and we ended up making out in that parking lot for a long time. I'm ashamed to say that the feelings I was feeling at that moment was not real love. It was immature, visceral, and very biological.

We drove back to the school, and she spent the night with me in my dorm room, curled together on my single bed. I didn't have a roommate currently, so no one was there to hear the secret whisperings between us late into the night.

When Ruth flew back into Amarillo, I was there to pick her up. I was confused about how I felt about Victoria, and I felt like I was staying true to my word to Victoria, when we had talked about being married soon, and spending our lives together.

I asked Ruth if she would drive out to our spot with me. She quickly agreed, and I could tell that she was massively nervous. I drove out on the dark back road to Palo Duro Canyon. There was a turnaround spot on that dark road that we had stopped at several times during the previous summer. It became "our" spot. It was on top of a gentle rise, and you could see all the lights of Amarillo down in the valley below the parking spot.

We got out of the car, and just enjoyed the quiet of the fall night. It was a little chilly, but the winds were calm for once, and we could talk quietly if we wanted. Eventually I turned to her and told her that I was ready to make my decision, but I wanted to do something first. I look back on my immature 18-year-old self in that moment and know that what followed was the wrong thing to do. But in the moment, I felt so right. I told her that I wanted her to kiss me. She had never had a kiss from a boy before, and it would be her first. I knew the importance of this, but I wanted to make sure that I was making the right decision. She was extremely nervous but went against her faith and better judgement and allowed me to kiss her.

Her lips were soft and felt good. But it was awkward and didn't taste like what I thought it should. In my mind, it didn't feel right at all. I did not consider this was her first experience kissing someone else. I didn't consider how I was stepping on her faith and vow to Jesus to wait for marriage for any kind of physical intimacy. I didn't see how selfish I was behaving. I just felt that this kiss would tell me everything I needed to know, and I was disappointed. The romanticized sparks didn't fly like I thought they should. I know now, at the age of 40 that the real connection with a woman is the trust and realization that she sees you for who you are and pushes you to be a better man.

There were a thousand other ways to know that Ruth was the woman for me, but I ignored them all, and used that kiss as the basis for what I did next.

I broke her heart into a million pieces when I told her I was going to marry Victoria. I crushed her spirit, and I don't know the emotions she went through for days to come, because when I dropped her off at her house, feeling excited that I was going back to school to tell Victoria what my decision was, I didn't see the look she gave me. I didn't feel the loss and heartbreak she did. And she never spoke to me again.

That night, with that awkward kiss, I lost the only real love I had experienced since my father passed away. I threw away a life that could have been everything I dreamed about my whole life.

And my justification was the physical activities that Victoria would do with me, and I knew I would have had to wait for Ruth to be ready for.

She was pure, and I felt like I was trash.

I lost her forever. It would be years before the impact of this would bow me under, and the knowledge of how I hurt her would crush me when I looked at where my life was, and where it could have been.

I married Victoria, against all advice, three months later.

Chapter 12

Many things seemed to happen all at once during those three months between choosing Victoria over Ruth, and us getting married on a cold, bitter, overcast Saturday in January. The biggest thing is Victoria and I decided together to drop out of school.

We thought we could just get jobs, and we would be happy. Life hit us hard. We learned that we didn't have good credit established, so it was near impossible to find a nice apartment, and the jobs we thought were abundant, just weren't there. We found a little apartment that I paid for six months in advance from an inheritance my aunt and uncle had built up for me.

They had been taking my social security checks every month while I was at Boys Ranch and putting them in a money market account for me. It was supposed to be for a down payment on a house eventually, but I got ahold of the money and blew through it rather quickly. Victoria helped considerably with that, but the end of the day, it was my decision, and mine alone, and I let my aunt and uncle down by how I treated what they had saved for me for so many years.

I came to realize a very important distinction during this time in my life. I learned that I lamented so much from so many years of things being done to me, which was out of my control. Obviously, my childhood still affected me, but I have no one to blame for how I allowed it to skew how I saw the world, or the needs I felt I had to have met at the time.

I learned that then, as a young adult, I oversaw my life, and I was making decisions based off reactions to the world, and what it did and didn't give me. I was very immature, trying to act like a grown up. Victoria and I were so young at this time, and we made so many bad decisions. Leaving school, moving in together, getting married so quickly, and the career choices I made in those early months of our marriage, were all decisions we should have made differently.

By Christmas of 1997, I had officially proposed to Victoria in front of her entire family, and my brother. We had driven my new car up to Great Lakes, Illinois, near Chicago, to pick my brother up from "A" school in the Navy and bring him back to Texas for the holiday. It was a great road trip, and I learned how much I loved driving long distances like that. We spent time with both of our families, and I could tell even then that no one was happy about where Victoria and I were. We should have stayed in school. We were working dead end jobs in Amarillo. She was folding and stocking clothing at a Target, and I worked dayshift at a telemarketer firm, selling America Online subscriptions and upgrades. AOL is now defunct, but at that time, they were the largest online provider in the country. I made medium wage, and so did Victoria. The only caveat at the time is that we did not have children yet.

My family and friends were still harboring anger at me for how I had treated Ruth. Everyone, including the Staff family, and my aunt and uncle had loved Ruth. I was making daily bad decisions, and I wouldn't listen to any of them. Victoria and I were going to the church I had gone to with the Staff family in Amarillo, and I asked the leader of the young adult's bible study if he would marry us.

His name is Jud Wilhite, and he is a nationally known pastor out of Las Vegas now, and I hear his messages every day on K-Love radio station. When I knew him in Amarillo, he was married to his wife, Lori, and they made an amazing couple. Jud has always been one of the smartest, well-read men I knew, and his faith is apparent in everything he does. I have read his books now and am impressed with him even more than I was twenty years ago.

On January 24, 1998, Jud married Victoria and me in a small gathering room in the large church in Amarillo. Victoria's sister, Tonya was there, as well as two friends of ours. No one else in either of our families would come to our small wedding. That night, we were at her parent's house, as she had a small bridal shower with the women from the church she grew up in, in Plainview, Texas. We made love that night, and 40 weeks later, our first son, Graham was born.

There is one situation that needs to come to light from the time between dropping out of school and getting married. Victoria and I were living in our one-room apartment in Amarillo and working low paying jobs. We had an apartment full of furniture we had on credit, and we thought we were grown up. On this evening, we were both home from work, and I was cooking dinner.

Victoria came into the small kitchen, and there were, again, tears in her eyes. I had music playing, so I turned it down, and asked her what was wrong. She didn't want to tell me at first, but eventually she got the whole story out.

She asked me if I remembered her high school friend who had come to our apartment about a month and a half before this evening.

His name was Cy, and he showed up one evening with a mutual friend of Victoria's. We invited them in and visited with them late into the night. I had to get up early the next day, so I told Victoria I was going to bed. I bid her friends good night, and trusting in her completely, I went to sleep.

A month and a half later, she is standing in our tiny, white kitchen with hamburger helper cooking on the stove and told me what she had been doing in the meantime.

It seems that the guy I had met, Cy, was not just a friend. He was her first boyfriend, and they had been inseparable all through high school. They had a messy breakup when she moved to Canyon for college but had seen each other every time she went back to Plainview.

When she and I started dating, she called him and told him. But seeing him again that evening in Amarillo, at our apartment that I had paid for, brought back so many feelings for her.

Apparently, that night, after I went to bed, the other friend left, and Victoria and Cy were alone. They were physical with each other that night but didn't go all the way to sex. But she went to Plainview almost every weekend after that night to see her parents. She explained that her parents were having some health issues, so she was going back on the weekends to help them.

Apparently during these visits, she would see Cy, and they would have sex. Every single weekend. I had no idea, and the trust that I had for her evaporated as she told me, in our kitchen, six weeks later.

I had a decision again to make. I thought back over what I had done to Ruth, and those doubts started creeping into my mind. We talked long into the night, and she promised she would never cheat on me again and would cut Cy out of her life completely.

I eventually believed her and told her I would still marry her the next month, and that I still loved her.

I was heartbroken and started feeling those feelings of mistrust I had had so strongly as a child. Outwardly, I acted like everything was ok between us, but I hated her, and hated myself for choosing her over my best friend. My insecurities and fear of being alone led me to still marry her and stay with her through many more painful times in the years to come. Painful times that we inflicted on each other.

At this point, I needed to make a drastic change in our circumstances.

I made a career choice, and it changed the direction of our lives, once again.

I enlisted in the military.

I visited with each of the recruiters for the different branches of service, and the Air Force was the only branch which made me feel like I had to be good enough to join them. The rest would take me in a heartbeat. I had a great ASVAB score from high school, and I was top 10% in school. I was fit, in great shape, and very smart. I wanted to be Special Forces, and the Air Force Special Forces were some of the most elite.

A lot of people aren't aware that the Air Force has Special Forces.

PJ's and CC's are the top of the game. I wanted to be one. I took all the tests to qualify for the PJ's program and passed every one of them.

I went into the service guaranteed Special Forces, but my uncle Travis had some very sobering advice for me. I went to him with the news that I was going into the Air Force, as he had retired from the Air Force years prior. He was happy for me but told me to get to basic training and ask one question about my new job. He told me to ask them what the TDY rate would be when I got to my first duty station. TDY is the Air Force acronym for being deployed.

When I got through the first part of basic, and they take you into an office, so you can sign your contract for the guaranteed job you asked for, I asked that very important question. How much would I be deployed?

These guys must be honest with you, unlike recruiters, and they told me very bluntly that I would be deployed at least 6 to 9 months out of the year for the first five years.

I would be places I couldn't tell my family where I was, and while Special Forces put on rank quickly, it was still a long way to go before I was high enough rank that I could choose how much I deployed.

Well that was not good news. I was newly married, and she was five months pregnant. I had not seen her for the five weeks I had already been in basic, so I couldn't see myself being gone that much.

So, I asked what other job they could offer.

They scrambled and looking at the fact that I scored the highest in Mechanics on the ASVAB, they offered me the job of Jet Engine Specialist.

I signed on the dotted line for six years of my life, and after basic, off to Jet Engine school I went.

I had no idea that this choice would, again, affect and change the next 22 years of my life.

Chapter 13

There were so many other, important things happening in my life at that time. I haven't discussed Basic Training, and how hard it was. I haven't discussed how Victoria's mother had complete kidney failure while I was in San Antonio, at Lackland Air Force Base for basic, and how Victoria wasn't able to write to me during the time her mother was in the hospital.

I received a package on my 19th birthday, while in basic training, and I saw that she had tried to write me every day. She was good about making me feel loved while I was away.

She would put her favorite lotion on the letter tops. It was White Gardenia, and the smell associated her pregnancy in my mind.

I loved her the most when she was pregnant. It was such an awesome time to be with her and see her growing belly.

I learned we would be having a son. We threw names back and forth for a long time, but finally settled on a re-spelling of the last name of one of her friends in high school.

Graham Connelly would be born in October 1998, very soon after I got to my first duty station in Oklahoma City, Oklahoma.

Tinker Air Force Base, home of the 552nd AGS. The squadron for the fleet of AWACS the Air Force had in operation.

I was to break my teeth on the TF-33, a Pratt and Whitney engine that had seen years of service on platforms like the B-52's and the widely used refueler, the KC-135. It was a solid engine, and I enjoyed my job of troubleshooting, fixing, and operating it.

Being in the military is difficult, but if you enjoy your job, it makes it tolerable. The worse part about my squadron, is that it had the highest operational rate in the Air Force. I was told my first day in the shop that within six months to a year I would be deploying to the Middle East, and to expect to do that two or three times a year.

Deploying was not the hardest part of this time of my life. When Graham was born, I was both excited and scared. I learned the first time that I held him that I would make a great father. I wasn't nervous of the messy part of having a baby. When the nurse asked me to help her bathe him for the first time, I held him with such confidence that it surprised me, and the nurse as well.

She commented that I was a natural, and I was so proud of that.

Victoria had had a difficult delivery. She was a little thing to begin with, and Graham was a monster of a newborn. He weighted right at nine pounds and was nineteen inches long. I called him my little Butterball.

The only doctor we could find on such short notice after moving to Oklahoma City was an older man on the last legs of his career. When Graham was being delivered, the doctor decided to use forceps on him, which bruised his little face, and Victoria ripped instead of having the surgical episiotomy, so her recovery time after delivery was intense.

Back at the townhouse we had moved into, she was unable to walk up the stairs to our room, or Graham's newly furnished nursery. She had to sleep downstairs on the pull-out couch for two weeks. She didn't get to see Graham sleeping in the crib that she had slept in as a baby for the first time. She could barely walk. It was a significantly hard time for her, and I did everything I could to ease the burden, and at the same time, get acclimated to my first military assignment.

Luckily, Graham was a very easy baby. He started sleeping through the night early on. He was being bottle fed, as Victoria was not able to breast feed. I think in a way she was upset about that. But she had tried to get him to latch on at the hospital to no avail. We were under the poverty line, with me being a low-ranking new troop in the Air Force, so we were fortunate to be on WIC, and got Graham's formula for free from the state. That was a huge blessing. His diapers almost bankrupted us, though.

Graham's first day home, he slept on my chest as we watched as the 49ers played the St. Louis Rams, and defeated them 28-10.

They went on to play in the playoffs that year but lost one game before the Super bowl. It was a great season, and I loved being able to watch some of the games with my new son.

Of course, he didn't know he was watching his father's and grandfather's favorite team, but it's the spirit that counts.

I was only 19 years old, so was unable to go to a sports bar to watch the games, while drinking a beer. Here I was, a new father, and I wasn't old enough to drink a beer. I could barely vote.

I still feel to this day, that new fathers that young do not have the abilities or resources, typically, to handle a new baby. If I could teach my sons anything later in life, it was to live their lives as long as they can before having a child. You must learn how to lose your selfishness when you have a baby. Nothing is about you anymore. It's all about the baby. And it should be that way.

I learned something about myself during this time. I loved being a father, but I was not very good at it. I got frustrated every time Graham cried. Later in life, and many children later, I would get to a point where a crying baby was a sweeter sound to me, but in those early days, I couldn't handle it sometimes, and often had to leave the house and take a walk when he was inconsolable.

Victoria was a great mother during those times. She had to take a lot on herself, as my shift seemed to change all the time. I would work dayshift for three months, and then they would send me to night shift. Many nights, she had to handle Graham alone. I think we made it work, but it was very difficult. Victoria's mother, Judy, was a huge help. She had run an in-home daycare for many years, so was an amazing resource for help.

We struggled financially during this time, as many young couples do. But we could never get ahead. We would carry over bounced checks from one paycheck to the next, and along with the penalty fees, could never seem to get out of the hole. When tax time came around, we spent our returns on things we needed, like a car, or furniture. We started out with very little. Very, very little.

Later, I would study Maslow's hierarchy of needs. Victoria and I, for our entire marriage, would never get off the bottom of that pyramid. We struggled to survive, and to feed the kids, and pay the rent. We could never save any money, and it took a toll on our relationship.

There has only been one period of my life, so far, where I didn't struggle every day.

During the first 40 years of my life, I spent a whole lot more days with no money in my pocket, than days with money.

The kids were always fed, and clothed, and went to school every day, but it was a struggle to have anything extra, and it kept me up many nights.

I felt in my soul that I had a purpose, as well as a potential that I wasn't meeting. Those two things drove me crazy as I tried to rub two nickels together most days.

There were periods where I would work 8 to 10 hours overnight on base, only to get home at 7am, and Victoria would be leaving for her day job.

I would have to stay awake and watch the baby. When Victoria got home from work in the late afternoon, I would finally be able to sleep for a couple of hours before I had to go in for my next shift.

It was a grueling existence, and I started to feel a bitterness creep into my spirit. I would pray to God, but I felt like He did not hear me.

I had yet to give my life to Christ, but why didn't God care about me in those days?

This theme would stay in my mind for a long time, and the negative feelings I would have for God intensified my depression.

When Graham was 7 months old, I deployed for the first time to the Middle East.

I was gone for six months, and my marriage would be stretched like never before.

Chapter 14

When you deploy overseas, the military tries to get you and your family as ready as possible. There are many briefings, as well as information given to your wife about services she can take advantage of while the service member is away. All this helped us prepare for my being gone for an extended amount of time.

The war in Iraq was in a standstill in 1999, but Operation Northern Watch and Southern Watch were in full swing. We were sending squadrons of jet fighters and bombers fully loaded everyday into Iraq, and they were coming home empty, every day.

At that time, Saddam Hussein was still in power, but not for much longer. I was deploying to Incirlik Air Base, near Adana, Turkey. It was very near the Syrian border, so it was considered a war zone, and we were heavily briefed on the culture, as well as the danger we were in, by being "in-country".

I was very nervous but was more nervous about leaving my wife alone back home. I would later learn that she wasn't always alone during this time.

Victoria and Graham went with me to the airport in Oklahoma City, and we said our goodbyes. They were tear-full, and sad, but I knew I was doing a good thing for my country and was excited to see some of the world.

On the trip over the pond, we would be stopping in England, Germany, Italy, and finally, into Turkey. I was finally going to see the world.

But I was very sad to leave my family behind. I knew that Victoria could handle things while I was away, but I worried about her being alone. I knew she didn't do well by herself. She would get lonely and sad. I worried, as all married service members do, about her cheating on me.

There were so many stories floating around the shop about married guy's wives doing abject things while their husbands were deployed. We all worried about "Jody" back home. A "Jody" was a civilian or military man back home who would woo our wives and girlfriends, and who would take our places in our beds with them.

This time away would test our commitment to each other, as well as stretch our devotion to our vows. A test we would both fail.

Being in other countries was an amazing experience. The best part was the food. I especially loved Turkish food. It was so clean and differently spiced. I learned that I'm a bit of a foodie. I loved trying the different foods from different countries. I had amazing sausage in Germany, and the best pizza and pasta I've ever had in Italy. We were only near the military bases, but even so, I felt like I got a taste of the region.

Traveling around the world gave me a bug to do more of it whenever I got the chance.

I also learned how much the rest of the world detests Americans.

As a country we have our own identity, but it's made up of being a hodge-podge of other cultures. All around the world, they have ancient customs and traditions that we could never mimic here in the US. We just haven't the longevity as a country. The rest of the world sees us as the accidental youngest child born to older parents, with older children, who all despise the youngest. It's a terrible analogy, but apt.

When I arrived in Turkey, it was night time. It was brutally hot, and the air felt wrong. It wasn't clean at all. I would later say to other's who have never been there, that the land was all used up. The dirt was not the fertile brown soil I was accustomed to back home. It was practically sand, and very few things grew there. The people were poor but didn't seem to know it.

We had been briefed on the cultural niceties we had to observe. Being left-handed was difficult because in public, in Muslim societies, it was offensive to do anything with the left hand. Also, the men were especially affectionate with each other, but the women were shunned in public. All these differences in society were things we, as Americans, had to accept and get used to. Which was fine. I never had a problem acclimating to other cultures. It was a lot of fun.

The job itself in Turkey was hectic. We were working 12-hour shifts, 7 days a week. I barely had time to myself after work. My sleep cycle was off because of the time difference. But overall, except for the problems back home, it was an amazing time to be overseas. I loved the experiences of seeing parts of the world that most Americans would never get to see. I especially enjoyed one tour I took of the bible regions of Turkey.

Tarsus was where the Apostle Paul was born. The Cappadocia region was spoken as one of the 12 churches of the New Testament.

Seeing all these regions of an age's old country was the highlight of my life. If only I hadn't learned what my wife was doing while I was away.

When I deployed to Turkey, Victoria drove Graham 6.5 hours away from home and left him with his grandmother in Plainview, Texas. A small West Texas town that I grew to hate.

I knew she was going to do this but didn't know the repercussions of it.

Graham spent the next couple of months with his grandmother, Judy, and Victoria went back to Oklahoma City, basically feeling like a single girl.

106

She met an enlisted Navy sailor and started a relationship. I found out about it by talking to her on the phone one day and hearing my front screen door open, over the phone. It was rather loud, and I hadn't gotten around to oiling the hinges while at home.

I asked her who had come into the house and she told me it was one of her girlfriends. I was weary, so asked if I could talk to her girlfriend, and she quickly had to get off the phone. I didn't trust her, so called back a couple of minutes later and insisted on talking to her friend. She broke down and informed me it was not her girlfriend who had come in, and after a long conversation, I found out that she had been spending the nights with this man she had met at her job. They had apparently been spending a lot of time together, and obviously I wasn't happy about it.

But I had my own secret. I had met a girl in Turkey, who was in the Marines, and who had been from Romania. Her name was Mireala. We had been having a month-long affair.

She knew all about my wife. I was never secretive about it. So, Victoria and I had both found comfort with other people.

Our marriage would survive this new encounter, but it would not survive much longer after all the others. We got married young, for all the wrong reasons, and obviously were neither ready for it.

I came back from deployment early, after my command learned about my wife's affair with the other married service member. He got in a lot of trouble with his command, and the Air Force brought me home early to see to the affair, and to get my household in order. They offered help with divorce proceedings and gave me all the support I needed.

When I got back to the US, and a guy in my shop picked me up from the airport and dropped me off at my house, Victoria and I reconciled, and decided to keep our marriage going. We made love that night like we hadn't in a long time. She was wearing a silk nightgown I had bought her in Turkey and sent home a month earlier. She looked beautiful, and I had missed her immensely.

Nine months later, our second son, Channing Blaine, would be born. We spent the pregnancy getting re-acquainted with each other, and trying everything we could, alone, to make our marriage work. Again, she was pregnant, and I loved her the most when she was pregnant. It was a happy time for us as a family, and looking back, I felt it was the best time. We also decided after Channing was born to open our marriage. We both wanted to experience sex with other people, and we decided, if we did it together, it would be ok.

I can tell you, for me, it was not ok. It ultimately destroyed our family. There was one particular time, after we allowed a stranger to come into the sacredness of our already broken marriage, we were in our bedroom, and I looked at her face, and then at the stranger standing behind her, having sex with her, and I could honestly feel my mind detaching.

She was no longer the woman I loved.

But it was my fault. I wanted her to not hurt me or leave me so much, I allowed my base, core beliefs to be torn to shreds.

From that day on, I no longer thought the same way about my marriage. There was no more hope. No more pureness. I was sickened that day, like I had been as a child, laying in the evening dusk, the shadows lengthening, and listening to the sounds of pleasure coming from my mom and the guy she replaced my father with.

Those feelings, that sickness in my soul, would change my decision-making ability for many more years to come.

We lasted four more years together, and while rocky, and very tremulous, it was a lesson that would last with me for the rest of my life.

It was a lesson I would use to have the strength to leave unhealthy relationships in the future.

I learned mistrust like it was a second skin.

And at the end of our marriage, Victoria, too, would leave me, with my children, just like everyone else had done through my life.

It became a pattern that would last until it didn't anymore. And I became the one to leave before they could leave me. I would rather run, then face that pain from then on.

When I got back from that deployment, one other thing happened that affected me for some time. I received a package in the mail from Mireala.

She had sent me a book I had never heard of before, but which opened my eyes to the types of books I would later come to love. The book was called "Love in the Time of Cholera" by Gabriel Garcia Marquez.

She had included a hand-written note, and two pictures of her taken in Romania. I remember in one, a Polaroid, she was picnicking in front of Dracula's Castle. I won't summarize the book here, but it changed my idea of what love was. It completely changed it.

To this day I think I loved Mireala. It was short, sweet, intense, and very real. I sometimes wonder what ever happened to her. She wasn't like anyone I had ever met before, but she opened my eyes in a lot of ways.

The whole experience of being in another country and seeing a lot of the world really woke me up to the fact that I had been fed a single story of the rest of the world my whole life.

There is so much more out there that we as American's don't realize. The world is as rich, and vibrant, and colorful as we think we are here in the U.S.

Other countries have a history and culture we have no idea about. They find importance in things we do not.

I think I'm sometimes sad that we have isolated ourselves in this country. We think we are superior, but we really are not.

The rest of the world has a vibrancy that we could only hope to one day achieve in this country. And that's what led to my love of traveling as much of it as I could.

Chapter 15

For four years active duty Air Force, I deployed five times. Each time was difficult, and I lived in a constant state of fear for my marriage.

The emotions I felt hovered around thoughts like, "I'm not good enough." "There's someone better." "What have I done wrong?" Those self-defeating feelings really put me into a depression. I did not like my job anymore and looked for any way to get out of the service.

I had changed jobs while in the Air Force, going back to what I had wanted to do in the beginning. Being deployed was scary, but not like I thought while at basic training and looking at it as it pertained to my newly growing family.

Now, I was fine being gone as much as possible, and it really strained my marriage even more. And then I was injured while being deployed.

I won't speak of that time. Maybe one day I'll be able to talk about it. But not today.

After, I just wanted to go to college and try to live up to my potential. Living up to my potential became a mantra for me.

At the time, I was nearing my mid-twenties, and I felt like I had accomplished very little in my life. Many would say that I did a lot. I had traveled all over the world, working for the military. I had been married for five years and had two sons. But I just didn't feel like I had done what God put me on this planet to do.

I tried to supplement my growing unease with being involved in our church. I worked as a youth leader, mentoring the newly put together band made up of youth from the church, and I actively participated in many aspects the church put together. But even that didn't satisfy me. I was growing quite restless with my life. I felt like I really needed to get back into school, and start learning something that would interest me, and which I could do something with.

Finally, the day came that my enlistment ended. I still had to serve in the reserves, but I was done being an everyday warrior, and I was happy to become a civilian. We were still in Oklahoma City, but when I asked Victoria where she wanted to go, she said she really wanted to go home to Plainview, Texas.

I knew that there was a college there, so I agreed. I felt it would be good for us to be back around her family, and the support would be nice. I wanted to use my GI Bill to go to school. So, scrapping together the money to move back to Texas, we loaded up the boys, and a large U-Haul truck, and headed west.

Arriving in Plainview, we had already arranged a rental home near where Victoria's mother lived. The plan was for me to get a job while Victoria watched the boys at home during the day. Almost immediately I got a job at a farm and ranch retail store. With my experience with horses and tack, and training, I was able to get that job easily. Fresh out of the military, I found that work was easy to come by. I also started helping Victoria's father, a man named Willie, who never had liked me. But he needed help, and I was in town. He ran the shooting sports team in the local 4H, as well as ran a trap shooting range. He had previously owned a gun store and indoor shooting range, so guns and everything gun related were in his wheelhouse in a major way.

Graham was, by that time, four years old and Channing was a bumbling two. They were beautiful little boys, and they thrived being around so much family.

Victoria's extended family were all around Plainview. Her grandparents were still alive, although getting older, and lived within ten minutes. I knew the boys needed this support of her family and found their identities in it. I never felt like I belonged though. Her family were good people, but they were not very welcoming to an orphaned boy from California, who aspired to a college education. None of her family made it past high school, and many not even that far They were just good southern people.

It took about a year to finally start college at Wayland Baptist University. Almost immediately I felt like I belonged. Here were people who were pursuing higher education, and I loved the challenges of learning new things and new concepts and excelled in class. I joined study groups and thought the deep thoughts encouraged in college.

I'm not sure how Victoria felt about me being away from home so much with classes, work, study groups, and school events. After we had been in Plainview for six months, she became pregnant again, with our third child.

Halfway through the pregnancy, we found out it was going to be another boy. That was three boys. My brother, at this time, had had two boys with his wife, and my sister, Venus Layne, had had three boys as well. Boys ran in my family.

It would be years before my parents, if they had been alive, would have had a granddaughter.

I'm sure you're wondering at this juncture in life, what became of my biological mother.

During my first two years in the military, Jasper and I had tried everything we could to find our biological mother, Margrit.

113

We found out that after New Jersey, she had moved with the two younger kids down to Punta Gorda, Florida. After further digging, and with the help of one of Jasper's friend's father, who was an FBI agent, we found out that Margrit had passed away in 1993.

We had no idea, for nine years by this time, that she had passed away.

Now we were truly orphans.

We had no way of knowing what had become of our younger siblings. Later, we would learn that they were put into the Foster Care system.

Little Edward was adopted by his foster family, but Venus Layne had a much harder road. At 16 years of age, and after being in the foster care system for years, she got into trouble with the law. She wound up in prison at 17 for four years.

In 2004, my mother's sister, Michelle, found me living in Plainview. She had seen some of my articles I had written for my college's newspaper. My first paid writing gig.

They were posted online under my name, and using some further sleuthing, found my phone number. The day she called my house on campus, Victoria answered the phone.

I had been at basketball practice. She was still on the phone with my aunt when I returned home.

I got on the phone, and my aunt was crying. She told me she had been looking for Margrit's four children for years. She had a vague idea where we had all ended up, but had not had any luck finding us, or contacting us, until she read my articles online.

We spoke for hours and hours, and I learned all about my mother's family, who all lived up near Boston.

I now had grandparents, aunts and uncles, and cousins. I was ecstatic. Here, finally, was my family.

I was able to travel to Boston on a couple of occasions to visit everyone. I looked like this family and was enveloped with love and acceptance.

It was a little strained with my grandparents because of their ideals concerning my father, which I felt were unwarranted, but which I understood, as he had been older than them when their daughter married him.

They had never approved of the union, and still didn't, 25 years later. But here was my family.

I would visit them several times over the next couple of years. But like everyone else, my grandparents would pass away within a couple of years, and when I eventually moved to Maryland, I would lose touch with the family except for the occasional phone call, or text during the holidays.

I still stay in touch with my aunt Michelle, but it's all so strained now. And after my youngest brother, Edward, would die in a tragic motorcycle accident, it all became so much harder to talk to each other.

I had also gotten back in touch with Linda, my step-mother, while I was in the military. She had stayed with Louie, marrying him, and they had lived together in Northern California. Being with him, she had lost all her children, and marrying him had stopped the social security checks from my father's death.

In 2001, Louie beat her up bad, putting her in the hospital. Zoie called me to tell me what had happened. Louie quickly went back to Hawaii, where he was from. Linda stayed in the hospital for a couple of months, and when the medical professionals saw that she was unable to care for herself, they put her into a nursing home at the age of 41. A year later, she would die of complications from her obesity.

The last time all five of us children were to be together was in 2002, at Linda's funeral.

I was fresh out of the military. Jasper was still active duty Navy. Zoie was starting her adult life and going to school.

Harmony, who had been adopted by a family in Lodi, was in Job Corp, which she would then have a career with as a teacher after graduation. Tony was a father and worked in law enforcement.

We gathered in the church that Zoie's adopted father ran and said our goodbyes to the only mother we had all known in early childhood. It was a very painful couple of days together, and emotions were so very high.

We promised each other to get together more often, but 17 years later, we still haven't all seen each other again.

For Jasper and me, we really were without parents of any kind now.

I flew back to Texas with a very heavy heart. We would all speak to each other on the phone from time to time, but the distances got further and further apart.

Zoie and Harmony still saw each other from time to time.

Jasper and I would have on again and off again contact for many years. We would eventually end up living together years later, but that was after so much more happening.

And all Tony would do is comment emoji on our Facebook posts. Whatever family we had once ended in 1988 when my father passed away.

In April of 2003, Riley Herbert was born in Lubbock, Texas. He was a beautiful and gregarious baby. As a toddler, he brought joy to my heart and laughter to his entire family.

Later, we would see the artistic soul he had, and encourage him with his gifts.

But by his second birthday, his mom and I would finally separate for good and get a divorce.

We did not end on a good note.

We had cheated on each other so many times, and ended up hating each other. It had been a mistake to have gotten married, and now there were three small boys who would grow up in a broken world because of us.

But I didn't know just how bad it would get.

The next four years, from 2005 to 2009, would be some of the most difficult years I would go through.

And at the same time, as you will see, my world would suddenly make sense, and I would find what it takes, in a solitary confinement jail cell in Vernal, Utah, to find peace at long last.

Chapter 16

Drinking alcohol, for me, had always been a social thing. Especially on deployments in the military. There had been so much drinking that I have no idea how anything ever got done. But we managed.

After my divorce to Victoria, I started drinking like it was my new job, and I had to excel at it at all costs. This habit got me kicked out of college and would basically be all I would do for quite a while. I moved into my own little apartment in Plainview, so I could still see the boys. Victoria moved in with her mother, and then eventually got her own little apartment. We stayed in touch for the boy's sake, but also because we were very co-dependent on each other, and tried to control each other.

She would get massively jealous of any girl I dated, and I would find out who she had been with from mutual friends, which would make me drink more. We both ended up working dead-end jobs at a local restaurant. So, now we saw each other every day at work, and I would watch as she would flirt with, and date, different people we worked with. She would watch me do the same thing. And date I did.

I started sleeping with any woman who would have me. I was 26 at the time, and I was dating and sleeping with 18-year-old college students. The main one at the time was named Tiffany. I think that in a lot of ways, I really messed her up. She may have been a tad bit broken when we met, but I used her so much, and in so many ways, I don't think she recovered for many years.

There was a boy who was in love with her for most of her young life, but she broke up with him to be with me. He came to the gym where I was working out one day while we were dating and asked me to be good to her. I couldn't believe this kid was telling me this, but I ignored it.

I was such a horrible person at that time.

She is now married to him, and they have a gorgeous daughter. I don't know that she's very happy, but she's content, and has a peace she didn't have when I knew her. She has battled cancer since then and shows how strong she is every day. Her husband, understandably, has many demons, and while I am not one to talk, or offer advice, still pray for their continued success and happiness. If anything, she has stability. She needs that as much as I do.

I would have parties at my townhouse where there was so much alcohol and weed that it would knock me out every night.

I was so mentally screwed up at that point. I didn't care what I did, or who I did it to, and it affected every part of my life. I had many jobs but couldn't keep one. I started hanging out with two specific guys that were just not good people. Eventually everything would catch up with me.

After a fight with these two guys, a warrant was issued for my arrest for Aggravated Assault with a Deadly Weapon, and Criminal Trespassing. I did what I had always done. I ran away from my troubles.

After Tiffany, I had been dating another 18-year-old student at Wayland named Sara. She was from SE Colorado, and the day I learned there was a warrant out for my arrest, we decided it was smart to head to her hometown.

While we were driving her car to Colorado, we decided that if I were going to prison for up to 20 years, it would be smart if we got married, so she could handle all my belongings.

This was such a bad mistake, but we talked her parents into it, and a week later, we were married in a small ceremony at the church she had grown up in.

A week after that, we went back to Texas at night and loaded up my furniture and belongings.

We moved to Pueblo, CO and started working. My college experience majoring in Psychology for two years landed me a job working with at-risk youth in a halfway house. Sara worked at a bank.

For six months or so we were poor and happy.

The law didn't catch up with me at that point, but I had also not seen my boys. I went down to Plainview once to pick them up and bring them to Colorado for a visit. It was a very hard two weeks, and I wouldn't see the boys for another year.

There was a lot going on in mine and Sara's lives at the time. I had so much pressure on me from running from my boys in Texas, as well as the law there. But there were a lot of good things as well.

Sara was young, yes, but she was very sure of her ideals about marriage, and relationships. I was in a place in my life where I didn't trust anyone, especially in a relationship. Sara took a lot of abuse from me because of my miss-trust, but also because I was still in a frame of mind of not caring about anything or anyone but myself. I was so damn selfish. Anyone else would not have stayed with me. I was a terrible person. I thought, incorrectly, that I was always doing the right thing, but the truth is, my viewpoint of life, and pretty much everything else was horribly skewed by this point.

But Sara was amazing. No matter what, she wanted to be by my side. She chose me over her family in a lot of ways. It may have not been healthy, but she had an amazing ideal of what a wife should be. She never gave up on me, even when everyone close to her told her otherwise. She lived in hotels with me while I worked all day, and she had to find something to do.

I can't imagine her days. But she always had a smile for me when I came home.

I was in a perpetual bad mood, and I took a lot out on her. None of it was her fault.

Years later, I would look back on my relationship with her and realize some very hard truths. Sara actually did love me. It was patterned after her strict Christian upbringing, and her ideals on marriage came straight from the bible, but it was love. I know that now.

The hardest truth is that I took advantage of that love and devotion. I corrupted Sara in ways that I'm sure any of her other relationships later in life had to pay for. To my eternal disgust, I took advantage of her devotion for me from a place of not caring. She has every right to this day to hate me with every fiber of her being.

But, she doesn't. She would never believe what I am about to say, but it's so true. Sara really is a pure spirit. She always has been. She was and is beautiful in so many ways. And horrible and incredibly stupid men have taken advantage of that fact, starting with me.

Looking back on our time together, I know it was tough. We didn't have any money most days. I was sending a lot of money for child support to Victoria. But we managed.

Another huge blessing in our lives, and which Sara has always had, were her parents. They were amazingly strong, Christian people. Like most people, they had their challenges, but the biggest lesson I learned from Sara's parents is to work as hard as you can through anything.

Both of Sara's parents had multiple jobs and ran a ranch. Her father was a professional roper, and her mother had no fingerprints because she had worked them off. Much of their wisdom that they imparted to me has stuck with me to this day. I thought I was raised with a strong work ethic, but both of Sara's parents put me to shame. I felt lazy next to them both. Today, I take a lot of pride in working harder than anyone around me. I wake up very early and go to bed late. I stay sharp, and always ready to take care of anything. I look down on people who don't wake up as early as I do or plan out work the way I do. But I know without a doubt that I am still nothing compared to Sara's parents.

They tried very hard to impart financial wisdom to me back then. I was given the job of being the head of my household. I never did a good job at that. But they tried. Very hard. They went against their beliefs and doubts for me many times. At first, I think they saw in me whatever Sara saw. I let them down, as I did so many others at that time in my life.

If they ever read this, I hope they know that their lessons, their example, did not fall on deaf ears. Like so many other strong adults throughout my life, I have come to realize that what they imparted to me was the absolute correct way to live. Unfortunately, I learned most of that too late.

After some time in Pueblo, I heard about jobs in the oil fields in Utah and decided to apply. With my maintenance background in the military, I was hired as a field mechanic for a Fracking crew in Vernal, Utah.

So, off to Utah went me and my new wife. Again, she stuck next to me through it all, staying by my side as was her place in the marriage. Her ideals for marriage was spot on, and again, I didn't appreciate it at the time.

Before we left Colorado, we found out that Sara was pregnant. I was very excited, but the troubles down in Texas hung over every happiness we could find.

Sara had actually been pregnant one other time, but since our blood types were opposite Ph, she lost that first baby very early. I'm not sure we even told her parents about it since we were not married at the time.

As the months progressively got colder in Utah, and we found whatever solace we could in each other, I knew that Sara was too young to understand where we were, and what was going on in the world. She was not ignorant, but I hid a lot from her. It was never a good, pure situation with Sara, and it was completely my fault. I gave that woman scars that I hope and pray faded over the years. I am so ashamed when I think back on my time with her. She deserved so much better. She still does.

On Valentine's Day of 2007, our son, J.L. junior, was born. It was snowing so much that winter in Utah, that Sara wasn't able to make it back to Colorado for her baby shower. The passes were closed for the winter and didn't open back up for a couple of months.

The night before Junior was born, which was a total surprise as he wasn't due for a few more weeks, Sara and I went for a walk, late in the night.

It had snowed all day, and the town was eerily quiet, as only it can be right after fresh snowfall.

As we walked those quiet, snowy streets, I felt a form of happiness. I remember laughing with Sara and appreciating what she was going though.

I wasn't a complete monster. I loved her, in my own way. She was wearing a white sweater and a heavy jacket. Her feet crunched the snow in heavy black boots. I remember holding her close so she wouldn't slip.

She looked up at me, and I saw the love in her eyes. I saw the devotion and care. And I was scared of it. I didn't deserve it.

I went to work the next day with plans for my wife and I that night. It was Valentine's Day, and I wanted to do something special for her.

Half way through the morning, working about 25 miles from town, I got a phone call from Sara that her water had broken in our kitchen. I jumped into my boss's car, as we carpooled to work most days, and hit the gas. I got about a mile down the road and took a turn too sharply, and ended up in a snow bank.

Luckily, me, nor the car, were damaged. Very shortly, a man with a truck and a chain came along and got me out. Bless that man!

I made it to the hospital, where my boss's mother had taken Sara and she looked so beautiful. In pain, but extremely beautiful.

Here she was, almost 19 years old, alone in a strange place, except for me, who didn't appreciate her like she deserved, and she didn't have one member of her family with her.

Her family was incredibly close, and she relied on them heavily. But she was happy. She looked content to just have me, and the start of our little family.

Again, I never deserved Sara. That evening, our son was born, and as he came into the world, I had Sara's parents and grandparents on the phone so they could hear his first cry. Which they did.

Two beautiful months later, I was arrested on my way home from work, and once again, I lost everything I had worked so hard to get.

That fateful day, April 4th, 2007, the law in Texas would catch up with me, and I knew I was toast. They put me in a solitary confinement cell in the Uintah County Jail for 30 days before I was extradited to Texas. It was in that little jail cell, which I was shut in for 23 hours a day, where I finally got to the bottom of the hole I had dug for myself.

After being there for three weeks, I was completely done. Sara had called me and told me that she would be seeking a divorce and had already moved in with a guy we had known in Colorado. Within two more months, she would be pregnant by this guy, and would marry him as soon as our annulment was finalized. I believed I would not see her, or our son, ever again.

At the annulment hearing, which I was a part of over the phone from Texas, I was persuaded to give up my parental rights over Junior. I agreed, and to this day, that decision has haunted me.

I have heard rumors that he isn't biologically mine, but I was there when he was born. I also did not want to believe the rumors, but it gave me the excuse I needed to feel some peace from the decision I had made.

I cared for him for the first two months of his life, and I gave up without a fight. I think everyone around me thought that it didn't affect me, but as you are soon to see, it affected me greatly.

I would, years later, hear from Sara again. Right after her next divorce. She apologized for what her and her family put me through, but it was too little too late. But looking back, I wish I would have done more. I wish I would have tried to help with her son.

I saw his pictures through the years on her social media. If he ever reads this, I hope that he knows I loved him. That I once again made the best decision that I could at the time, and with the circumstances as they were.

In Colorado, he was surrounded by her wonderful family. He would know love and acceptance. I banked on God watching out for him, and keeping him safe, as I wasn't able to.

I hope one day to be able to do more, and not a day goes by that I don't think of that boy. I think if I can give him anything, it would be this book, and one day, he may try to understand where he came from. If he even knows who he is.

I know in my heart that I was using those rumors as an excuse to make myself feel better. I failed that boy. One day, I hope soon, I can make up for the years he lost.

In that jail cell in Utah, it was the middle of the night. I was weeping for myself, and the predicament I had put myself in. I was facing up to 20 years in prison in Texas, I was all alone, and there was no one in the world who cared about me.

These were the thoughts screaming in my head.

I had been sobbing for a couple of hours when I decided I wanted to die. Apparently this had been a theme in my life so far.

Looking at the cell, I thought that if I stood at one corner, I could get enough of a running start to bash my head in on the opposite concrete wall. I got down from my bunk and laid down on the cold concrete floor.

I was in so much pain.

Every bad thing that had happened to me in my life was crowding for attention in my mind. I felt utterly and completely alone.

I've read that at times like these, where a person is at the end of their rope, is when God will intervene. I was praying, but I didn't know I was praying.

Laying on that floor, my stomach in knots and tears streaming down my face, I opened my eyes and saw something in the back corner under the bunk. I had spent three weeks in this jail cell and knew every corner of it intimately. But I didn't know what I was looking at.

I reached under the bunk; my tears temporally forgotten. I felt a book under my hands and brought it out. I had not seen this book before and didn't borrow it from the cart that came around once a week. I looked at the title. "The Purpose Driven Life." By Rick Warren.

It struck me as odd, because I had lamented for so long on what my purpose was in this world.

I flipped through the pages, temporarily forgetting my hours-long suffering. I landed on Day 14, and the title said it all. "When God feels Distant."

I read those six pages for day 14, and it changed my life, right then and there. I closed my eyes and gave up my life to Jesus.

I had been baptized twice before in my life, and thought that I had received the Holy Spirit, but in that moment, I knew that I had not really given up control before.

In that small, cold, distant jail cell in Utah, I gave my life completely to Jesus, and gave control to God. I felt a renewing of my spirit that I learned later was spoken about in the Bible.

From that moment on, I no longer craved alcohol. My mind shifted. I felt clearer than I had in so many years. I felt His Spirit fill me up and make it so that I was never alone again.

I knew things would still be difficult, and they would be for a long time, but at that moment I knew that God was in charge, and He had a plan for my life.

At that moment, I was no longer scared. It would take a lot more, later down the road, to really learn His plan for my life, but in that moment, at the age of 28, I was free.

That night, I slept like a baby for the first time in more years then I could count.

At that moment in my life, I felt at peace. Finally, at peace.

I later was extradited to Texas in the back of a van, chained at the waist and ankles like a murder suspect, but I didn't care.

I would get to Texas, and after 100 total days of being behind bars, I would be free of all charges. Every day was a miracle.

When I needed a job, it happened that day. When I needed food, God made someone feed me.

I would try to take control back from God from time to time, but I knew that he was moving me towards something great.

When I got out of jail, I was reacquainted with the boys. Their mother had met a man named David, and they were all living together.

The boys would grow up with this family for many years. I would end up clear across the country. I would lose touch with the boys for years, but I would find them eventually.

I would take Victoria back to court and get joint custody of all three boys. They would come out to the other side of the country to meet their other family many times.

But as I would learn, life is a process. It changes all the time and only God can see the beginning from the end.

Many more wonderful and horrible things would happen to me in the years to come, but through it all was one unshakeable fact: God was with me, and I was His.

Even when I eventually lost and re-found my faith, God would never leave me. He replaced all the things I had gone my whole life without.

He became my Father in so many ways.

He never gave up on me. And He still hasn't.

The work He started in me is still in work, and I'm still finding the purpose He has for me. I learned that He is incapable of failing me.

It's so easy to have real faith when you believe that one statement.

He is incapable of failing me.

I would test Him, and He would test me in the years to come.

My journey wasn't over yet, but it had begun in that jail cell late that hot summer night, when I learned that I wasn't alone anymore.

I wasn't alone anymore. For the rest of my life.

Chapter 17

I had a new lease on life. I was feeling joy I hadn't felt before. I have since read about those first days after receiving the Holy Spirit. It's really a blessing during an otherwise confusing time. Everything just seemed to work out for me. Even though I didn't have a car, or much money, God still saw to my needs.

I didn't know where the road led, but I was on it. I was changed so profoundly that I didn't even cuss when I spoke anymore. I stopped having sex with every woman who showed me any attention like I had spent two years doing. I didn't even feel like I needed a relationship at the time.

I had a group of friends, and I started going to church again. This time, though, the sermons, and the bible readings meant so much more to me.

It was personal now.

I had a thirst for the Word. I started reading every day. I would have the opportunity to share with other's what I had been reading.

I started listening to Christian music again. I know I aggravated a lot of my friends with my new-found spirituality, but I didn't care. I was on fire for the Lord. And I felt love from Him like never before.

In the beginning of our walks with Him, we need those feelings of closeness with Him to keep going. Later, when it feels like He's not with us anymore, or when it gets hard, we can look back on those first days and remember that He hasn't changed.

We have.

I was again living back in Plainview, where I had gotten out of jail. I was seeing the boys again.

I got a job maintaining walking-floor trailers. It wasn't a great job, but it fed me and paid the rent.

When the boys would come over on the weekends, I had a little efficiency that I rented. It was hard to come up with money to feed them, as half of my paycheck was going to child support.

And I had a lot of child support to pay. That wouldn't end for quite some time.

After a couple of months of living like this, I had a talk with God. I felt like I wasn't doing any good for the boys. I was there for them, but couldn't feed them very well, nor give them anything they needed. Everything went to child support.

I also knew that they not only had Victoria's extended family but were now a part of David's family. I had no family for them.

I was on fire for God, but life was still there, and still getting me down. I prayed to God for what I should do. I didn't like the answer, and I'm still not sure to this day if it was the right thing to do.

My brother had come to visit me during this time, driving with his family from where he was stationed in California, out to Patuxent River Naval Air Station in Southern Maryland.

He saw how I was living, which wasn't great, and it stayed with him. When he got to Maryland, and had been there for a couple of months, he had the opportunity to talk to one of the managers of a company that had a contract with the Navy to fix airplanes. He asked the manager what qualifications he was looking for in new hires and called me that night. He told me that there was a great paying job out in Maryland that I qualified for, and if I wanted to come out, I could stay with him until I got on my feet.

So, after a lot of prayer, I decided to get on a bus, and head east. I once again left the boys, but I felt like they were in better hands than what I could give them.

I knew that if I got to Maryland and did well, and the job did pay extremely well, I could bring them out there and we could be together as much as I could get them.

I did not know, at the time, that Victoria would use that excuse to remove the kids from my life, and I wouldn't see them or talk to them for almost 6 years.

She changed her phone number, moved to a different house, and blocked me from all social media. I had no idea where they went, or if they were ok.

I constantly talked to the Texas Child Support people to send her word that I needed to speak to her and gave them permission to give her my contact information. I kept all the copies of the letters they sent her over the years and used that to gain joint custody later.

She even wrote my sister Zoie at one point and told her she wasn't going to give her any information on the boys because she didn't want it getting back to me. She now had her happy little family unit, and I wasn't there to disrupt it anymore.

It would be 6 years before I would see the boys again.

When I arrived in Maryland, I was in heaven. It was October, and it was starting to cool off. I was living in deep southern Maryland, near the Chesapeake Bay. The land was covered in woods, and I spent the first three weeks there walking in the woods and communing with nature.

I had spent so much time in the Texas panhandle, where there are no trees or water, that to be amongst so much beauty now was life changing.

I was also back living with my brother, who I loved so much. The mixture of communing with nature and being back with family was so good for my mental well-being. I was filled with the Holy Spirit and had not looked for any kind of romantic relationship with anyone for a good while at this point.

I was lonely, but I was ok with it. I wanted to find some way to get into some sort of routine, and just have some stability in my life for once. I felt like, at this time, the last twenty-nine years had been like a roller coaster, and I really needed to settle down.

I felt like Maryland would allow me to do that, somehow.

Within a couple of months of being in Maryland, my brother and I had a good group of friends, which we did everything with. We had weekly karaoke nights at an Irish pub. They would have our specific drinks ready for us when we got there.

Mine was a Black and Tan, and Jasper loved Yuengling. We would always start the night off singing "Save a Horse, Ride a Cowboy" by Big and Rich.

The pub was always full of regulars, and this became an integral part of our week. We also met for Saturday morning breakfast with the group at IHOP. And through the week we did various other things with different members of the group, but always were together.

I started working on base as a civilian contractor to the US Navy. I was making the best money I had ever made in my life. For once, I was content, but I didn't have the boys.

When I got settled into an apartment and had everything running smoothly, I tried to contact Victoria to see about flying the boys out. I wanted to take them to Washington DC and show them Southern Maryland. I wanted them to see the beauty in the world outside of the Texas Panhandle.

This is when I found out that I had lost every way to contact her. I sent letters that got returned, I tried to find phone numbers or email addresses. All to no avail.

Through the years I would do as many internet searches as I could. I would find an article here and there about the boy's achievements in school, so I was sure they were still in Plainview.

I didn't have the means to hire an investigator, or anything like that, and as time went by, I had the opportunity to begin things with who I thought was the perfect woman. Things got lost in the shuffle and routine of daily life. My work was demanding, my time spent with this woman started taking up more time, and the time with the group and my brother took up the rest.

I allowed six years to go by before I heard from the boys again. It was one of the saddest times of my life. I missed my sons. I missed them every day.

I felt like a failure, because here I was, sending bi-weekly child support payments that increased as my income increased, but I had no access to talk to, or see my boys.

They would grow up in their most important, influential years with another man.

With the success I was achieving in life, I felt like a complete failure to my children.

Chapter 18

When I moved to Maryland in 2008, my prayer life started changing. I had always said little, under my breath prayers, throughout the day, and I kept that habit going. I believed in the verses that told us to "pray unceasingly." I kept up a running dialog in my mind with God and would talk to Him like I would talk to a friend or confidant.

It kept me grounded, but it also made me feel less alone. I had good friends at this time, and a very supportive brother, but I lacked real love and commitment with a woman.

My second day in Maryland, my brother took me on base and while we were there, he introduced me to a woman named Priscilla.

Priscilla was apparently a big deal on base.

That's how she had met my brother. He was working for the Navy as a Health Inspector, and as such, had met Priscilla and showed her how and what he did in the inspections. Other than that, they had had no other contact, but he knew enough about her to know her name.

I was there with my brother when she walked inside the building we were in, and Jasper saw her and introduced us. I didn't really think much about meeting her, other than she was very attractive, but seemed stand off-ish.

She was pleasant enough, but it was a very quick hello, and she was off to do something in the building.

I remember commenting to Jasper that she was very pretty, and he said something along the lines of, "yes, but she's not very nice." I said, "I thought she was nice", and that was the end of the conversation.

Having a large group of friends that we hung out with all the time was so rewarding, but I also felt like I was missing something. I started visiting a couple of churches in the area, but as I was working very long hours, and it was very difficult work, I used my free time to sleep and go hiking.

I also got to know the area very well. I was living with my brother at his on-base housing, which I wasn't supposed to, and I needed to start looking for my own apartment.

One of our friends in the group was a woman named Vicky. She was active duty Army and performed the same kind of work my brother did on base. She was married, but her husband was deployed at this time, and she was actively seeking a divorce while he was away.

There was history of verbal and emotional abuse in the relationship, and she was very vocal about it. She was starting to stand up for herself and getting a divorce and moving on with her life was a great start for her.

We talked about how she had to move out of the townhouse she shared with her soon to be ex-husband and was looking for an apartment. I asked her if she would like to be roommates, and she agreed.

We started the search for a good sized two-bedroom apartment and found a great one rather quickly. It was close to the base, where we both worked, and had its own private beach, and was surrounded by woods. We put down the deposit, and moved her stuff in, little as it was.

At that time, since she had a truck and a horse trailer, she drove with me back down to Texas where my furniture was kept in a friend's garage. We picked up my stuff, drove back to Maryland all within a couple of days, and unloaded it at the new apartment.

All in all, we set up a rather comfortable living space. I would cook, and clean, and we both worked. She also had an amazing hobby.

She owned a horse, which was stabled nearby. She performed dressage at competitions and was always training and taking care of her horse. Since I had some horse training myself, I went with her to help, and picked up a part-time job at the stables she used, training, walking, lunging, and grooming horses there.

It was a nice little job that I loved doing.

So, I set into a routine. During the end of 2008 and the beginning of 2009, I worked the two different jobs, hung out with my group of friends, and basically kept to myself.

I still felt like I was missing something in my life, but I was happy and content.

Vicky and I soon started a physical relationship, but it was more out of shared loneliness and close confines in the apartment than a real relationship.

Basically, we slept together, but didn't develop feeling for each other. It was casual and convenient for us both.

The second week I lived in the apartment, I noticed something that would become very important later.

I was parking my car one evening and a blue car had followed me into the same parking area. This was weird, as the parking area for my building was way in the back of the complex and was quite secluded.

It meant that whoever was driving the blue car must have lived in my building. I got out of my car while the other person did, and I was shocked that I knew her.

It was Priscilla, the woman I had met on base several months prior.

137

I again noticed how attractive she was. I waved but I don't think she saw me. She walked up to the other staircase of the building and entered an apartment that was only two doors down from my own.

I didn't think too much of it at the time, but as the next couple of months would go by, I would start thinking about her more and more.

In May of 2009, it was starting to get hot. I made it through one Maryland winter and felt like I was ready for some warm weather.

The winter had been bad. We had a couple of snow storms, and a lot of wind off the Chesapeake Bay.

Working outside on the airplanes, it got to be miserable sometimes, but I still enjoyed my job. I got along with everyone, made some good friends, and felt like I belonged. I knew the lingo, I knew the work, and I was picking up certifications that would help me in my job. It was very satisfying work.

Towards the end of the month, Vicky and I had had some arguments. She was starting to feel feelings for me, and I wasn't interested in that at the time, at least not with her. She was a great woman, but her time and energy were spent all on her job and her horse, and there really wasn't the time left over for a relationship, or at least, the kind that I wanted.

We finally agreed that we were just going to be roommates, and nothing else.

On the 24th, I had been at the gym when I received a phone call. One of the other women in the group, Dawn, wanted me to go with her to get a pedicure. I had never had one, but agreed, as I hadn't seen Dawn in a couple of weeks.

I met her at the spa, still in my workout clothes, and we got the pedicures and chatted about life and work and other mundane things. I remember telling her though, that I was ready for a real relationship again.

It had been four years since I started divorce proceedings with Victoria, and I felt that I was ready to start again.

By this time, I really didn't even think about, nor acknowledge, the time I spent with Sara.

I didn't tell anyone that I had been married a second time, as there were no records of it. I pretty much wiped it from my mind.

I left Dawn at the spa and drove back to my apartment. I remember it was a Friday, and that weekend there was an airshow on base. One of our planes was on display during the show, and the Navy-Blue Angels were also going to be performing. I had watched them from the flightline at work all week practicing. I was very excited.

I pulled up to the apartments, and saw that the same blue car followed me in. I knew it was Priscilla, but I had not spoken to her in the months since I moved in.

I thought about her often though.

I noticed her medium length dark brown hair. I knew her eyes were dark brown like mine, and she was in great shape. I figured she ate well and worked out. She was tall. I thought about 5'7, which was nice.

Most of the women I had been with were short, and her height, and mind, made her seem very formidable.

She was one of the most beautiful women I had ever seen, and I would later learn that she knew that. She would show me a pride and a will as formidable as her looks.

I knew I was attracted to strong, driven women, but she was so much more than that.

I felt ugly next to her.

I didn't know what she would see in someone like me, but I also had sound confidence at this time, so I knew that if I showed her what I brought to the table, she would fall for me. I had little doubt that I wanted to date her.

But what I didn't see coming, was how much she would control every aspect of our eventual relationship.

But at the time, she was beautiful and enchanting, and enticing.

I wondered what she was doing in her apartment, and if she had a boyfriend. Every day when I got home, I would look at the windows of her apartment, and wonder if she was at home. I never had the nerve to knock on her door like I wanted.

But today would be different. I don't know if I was bolstered by the conversation with Dawn, or the pedicure made me feel attractive, or the stars aligned in a proper way, but at that moment, as I watched her park three spots down from my car, I was going to say hello.

She got out of her car, clearly just off work as she was wearing a white blouse with black slacks. I thought she looked very professional.

She pulled a sweater out of her car, and I would learn that she only wore black and white to work, and always had a sweater.

Very practical, and very boring. I would work on getting her to wear some color for many years.

I walked up on the sidewalk and as she turned towards the walkway leading up to her staircase, I approached and said hello. She returned the salutation.

"Do you remember who I am?" I asked.

"Yes, you're the health inspector's brother, what's his name? Jasper?"

"Yes, that's me. I saw a while back you lived here, but I didn't know if it was appropriate to say hello. I didn't know if you were single or with someone, so I never said anything." I stuttered, as I was getting nervous.

"No, I'm single, but I saw you, and thought you were with the woman who lives with you."

"No, we are just roommates."

"Well that's good." She said. "I had wondered how a woman like that was with a guy who looked like you."

At that, I knew that I should make the next move. She thought I was attractive, and I felt the same way about her.

"I have to go take a shower, and I'm walking in these paper sandals because I just got my first pedicure. But I want to keep talking to you. Are you busy tonight?" I asked, hopeful.

"No, I'm not busy. Why don't you come over after your shower and we can talk?" She said.

I had never taken a quicker shower, not even in Basic Training, where we only got two minutes to shit, shave, shine, and shampoo.

I dressed casually, as I didn't want to seem too forward. I didn't know if she would want to get food, or what. I sprayed on some body spray, hoping it wasn't too much.

Checking myself in the mirror, I thought back on her statement about me being good looking. I was excited to talk to her.

I walked down my stairs, went over to her stairs, and knocked on her door. She answered, and I saw that she had changed into a pair of jeans and a tank top. She invited me in, but I asked her instead if she wanted to go for a walk. She agreed, and locking her door, followed me down the stairs.

There was an amazing walking path around the neighborhood next to the apartment complex. It went through the woods, and was well lit. I had often walked the two-mile-long path and thought it a great place to walk with her. It was difficult not to notice how attractive she was. And as we talked, I saw she was very intelligent, well spoken, and highly educated. How is a woman like this single, I thought?

I came to find learn she had just graduated with her Masters. Getting her MBA helped her move up in her company. She was in line for a huge promotion that she was just interviewed for the previous day. I thought that was great. She started asking me pointed questions about what I did for a living, how much money I made, and what my goals and dreams were.

I answered all those as best as I could, and when she asked about dreams, I told her I had always dreamed of being a writer. She commented how that was a long way from being an aircraft mechanic. I said I know, but I have been working on airplanes for a long time, and sometimes I feel like I'm stuck doing that since that long-ago day when I changed my job in Basic Training.

As we walked, the overwhelming smell of the wild honeysuckle lining the path was very strong. We commented about it, and as time would go by, I associated that smell with her. Little things like that were always on my mind, and I knew things like that made me into a romantic.

We talked long into the night. We eventually ended back at her apartment. I was sitting on her couch, and she was in the chair opposite. We spoke about many things. I told her about my sons, and my previous marriage. She told me about her 7-year long relationship before she moved to Southern Maryland.

She was originally from Washington DC, and her parents still lived there. She had two older brothers, and one younger sister. As we got past midnight, I didn't want to ruin my welcome, so I told her I better go to bed soon.

I did, however, ask her if she wanted to go to the airshow with me the next day. She agreed, and we planned to drive together.

I told her I would call her in the morning to cement plans, and she agreed, giving me her number. I felt like it was too soon to try to kiss her, or even hug her for that matter. So, I told her goodnight, and walked back to my apartment. I stayed up late thinking about her, and the things she told me about her family. I felt there was a lot more there, and I was excited to learn all about her. I was a little smitten.

The next morning, I woke up early and went for a walk, as I usually did on the weekends. I smelled the honeysuckle again, and knew I had to call her. As I walked, I pulled out my cell phone and dialed her number, praying it wasn't too early. She answered and told me she had been up for a little while. A plan formed in my mind. I knew she had told me the night before that her favorite thing in the world was shopping.

She had worked retail at one time before moving up in that world. I told her I had a problem. I didn't have anything to wear to the airshow and wondered if she wanted to go to the mall with me to pick out an outfit. She agreed, and I told her I would be over to pick her up at 8am. The mall, which was about 50 minutes away, opened at 9am. She agreed, and I hurried home and showered.

Driving to the mall, we fell back into the same easy conversation from the night before. She was very classy. She wasn't like the women I had dated before. She was from the city and was very sophisticated.

It was 8 am on a Saturday morning, and she was wearing slacks and a blouse, her makeup perfectly applied to where it didn't look like she was wearing any. She had on an expensive perfume, which was very subtle, and she was just giving me a vibe that she may have been too good for me.

She was much more educated than I was, and I felt like, talking to her, she was more intelligent than me, but in different ways.

As we went shopping, she knew all the brands, and how things would fit me. I felt she was enjoying showing me her world.

I have never looked much into how a store is laid out, or how they display clothes. She explained all these things to me as we looked for an outfit.

I finally decided on a pair of nice khaki shorts, a blue button-down polo, and some soft deck shoes. I had never worn these kinds of clothes before, and I think she was getting a kick out of dressing a country boy from Texas who got his hands dirty everyday turning wrenches on airplanes.

Getting back to the apartment, I told her I would pick her up at 2pm for the airshow. In between getting back to the apartment, and picking her up, I called my brother and told him what had happened the last two days. He was excited for me but told me to be careful.

She had a reputation as being a real hardass. I could see that, as she hadn't smiled much during our time together, but I also chocked that up to it being a new thing for both of us, and we were both weary.

Taking her to the airshow was an amazing experience, until about halfway through the date. I was able to take her around to the various displayed aircraft and explain to her how things worked, much like she had explained things to me at the mall. I could tell she was impressed and asked quite a few questions about the planes. I shared my knowledge and felt like I was impressing her. All that changed as we walked over to find a seat to watch the Blue Angels.

An older man in a Navy uniform approached us and was saying "Hey Priscilla" as he drew near. I saw his rank on his collar and saw that he was a very high-ranking officer. He got close enough to shake my hand, and Priscilla introduced him as the Base Commanding Officer. They spoke pleasantries and he then invited us to sit in the VIP area for the flight display by the Blue Angels. To say that I was intimidated was a small way of putting it.

I didn't realize that with her new position, she was on the command board for the base. People knew her and knew who she was. She waved at several high-ranking people as we found seats in the Invitation-Only seating area.

I think she knew how intimidated I was and laughed at me. I shyly told her I was just a lowly contractor. She shrugged it off, and as we sat down, took my hand, and held it. This was our first physical contact. I felt very warm. We watched the Blue Angels perform, and I was explaining how Fat Albert, the Blue Angel's C-130 took off almost vertically with JATO rockets. She was impressed with that, and as I explained how I had been working on C-130's for a couple of months now, I knew all about them. Or at least I thought I did.

After the airshow, we didn't want to separate, so she asked me if I wanted to get dinner. I told her I did, but I wanted to go somewhere with her first.

Since moving to Maryland, my brother and I had been volunteering at a nearby national park for an event called "Vacations for Veterans". We basically worked with wounded veterans from the military hospital at Bethesda, giving them and their families a much-needed weekend vacation. All this took place at a park called Greenwell State Park, and it was here, and a certain spot, that I wanted to take her.

We pulled into the park close to twilight. I parked, and we walked down to a secluded beach next to the Patuxent River. It was a gorgeous night, and I wanted to make this perfect. I should have stayed with her on the beach, but there was a spot in the woods, with a little bit of effort and some hiking to get to, that I wanted her to see.

I took her hand and led her up the difficult trail to get to the top of the hill overlooking the beach. It was deep into the trees, but when we got to the top, a little sweaty, the overlook of the river and trees, and the beach, was perfect.

I turned towards her and told her that I had been in this spot before, and thought it was a great spot for a first kiss. I placed my hands on both sides of her face and brought her mouth to mine.

The kiss was sweet, and gentle, and was over very quickly. She was a little upset that she had gotten sweaty, and she said that she was getting eaten by the mosquitos.

So, what I thought was a perfect first kiss, she didn't like very well.

I shrugged it off and took her to dinner.

She was uncomfortable from sweating, but she was still pleasant to be around. I should have seen some red flags in this exchange, but I didn't care.

She was beautiful, and a little quirky. I learned she was not the outdoors type, and at the time, that was ok. I just really liked her.

Within three months, she would be pregnant, we would be living together, and I would have broken up with her three times because of her controlling, manipulative personality.

When I found out she was pregnant, I always came back. I wanted my child, much more so because by this time, I had lost contact with the boys, and I really wanted to be a father again.

I thought that I had been through emotional ups and downs before, but nothing that had happened in my life so far, prepared me for the next 10 years of my life together with Priscilla.

When I studied psychology at Wayland Baptist University, I had no idea some of those terms like Gaslighting, or Cognitive Dissonance, or the Cycle of Violence, would rear their ugly heads in my life.

But they did.

The core of who I was would be shaken, and it took everything I had to get out of it eventually, my body broken, my mind almost shattered, and my emotional state a complete wreck.

Finding myself after that would take so much more than myself, or any effort I did.

It would take a miracle from God.

Chapter 19

Prissy, as her family called her, got the promotion she had been trying to get. In late June of 2009 she was transferred to Washington Navy Yard for her new position in her company. Her new position would require her to travel to many bases from Washington DC to Maine, and the Chicago area.

She was gone two weeks out of every month, and it put a real strain on our relationship. By July 4th, we would break up for the first time. I didn't speak to her for three days, but we reconciled, and got back together.

In August, we decided, with her parent's blessing, to move in together, and we would do that in Waldorf, MD, because it was halfway between her new office, and where I worked at Patuxent River NAS.

By then, she had taken several pregnancy tests, which all came back positive. A blood test at her doctor's office confirmed it, and her due date was St. Patrick's Day, 2010.

The days started turning into fall. It started getting cooler, and the leaves on the millions of trees started changing colors.

This was my favorite time of year, and it was a special time in our relationship and time together. We were living in a very nice condo in Waldorf, which was newly built, and we were combining both of our salaries.

For the first time in my life, I could say that I was living a life that exceeded my expectations. We were both saving up money in retirement accounts and had extra every month to have lovely dates and eat at nice places. Prissy was accustomed to wearing expensive clothes and buying expensive makeup and perfumes. She got her nails and hair done as much as possible, and until our first child was born, we still maintained this level of living.

I bought a new jeep to drive, and she upgraded to a brand-new Honda, which had more room for the baby. We spoke about buying a house together, which was always a dream she had, but we didn't discuss marriage except maybe twice, and both times I told her that I didn't want to get married until I was free of debt and my credit was better.

My job working on military aircraft required a security clearance. I had been working on getting this clearance since I started the job, almost a year prior. I was doing everything they asked me to get approved.

I had to make sure the legal trouble I had had in Texas was all taken care of. I had to consolidate my debt into a government ran debt consolidation program.

We had the funds to do all this, but it took a lot of work.

Finally, right after my first daughter, Isabella Marie, was born in February, my security clearance came back approved.

I had worked under the knowledge that if it didn't get approved, I would lose my job, so there was so much stress over this the first year and a half.

But I could breathe again and focus on my new little bundle of girliness.

Halfway through the pregnancy, Prissy had a sub-chronic hematoma, meaning, Isabella had come a little unattached from Prissy's uterine wall.

She started bleeding very badly one night at home, and I rushed her to the emergency room. They said the baby was fine, but Prissy would need to be on bed rest for a couple of months.

Those were the hardest days for Prissy because she hated not working. She had worked so hard to get where she was, and being the first woman, and the youngest to get to that level, made her fiercely proud.

She had worked so hard to earn the three degrees she had. Two bachelors and an MBA. Lying in bed all day, with nothing to do, really got to her.

It was very difficult to handle her mood swings, but I also wanted my daughter to be born healthy, so I tried to make life as stress free as possible for Prissy. I know I didn't do a very good job of it, but I tried.

For Christmas that year, I was thinking long and hard on what to get Prissy as a present. I knew that she would be in bed for a couple of months, and then was going to take 6 months off when Isabella was born.

I remembered back to one time we had visited friends and played Wii bowling. I felt like she had had a good time, so I went to Walmart and purchased a Wii console.

When she opened it on Christmas morning, she was so disappointed, she made me return it.

She said I didn't know her at all, and I quickly found out that she wanted the same things for every birthday, anniversary, and holiday.

Some new pajamas, some perfume, a gift card to a spa for her nails or hair, and some expensive chocolate.

Until we finally divorced, I got her this exact same mixture of presents for every occasion. There was no change, and if I tried to surprise her with anything different, she made me take it back to the store.

Prissy started showing signs of Pre-eclampsia, so the doctors were very concerned about her blood pressure and made her stay on bed rest until the baby was born. I know at the time, I did not help with her blood pressure at all. I was still under strain about the security clearance, and dealing with Prissy's moods was taking a toll on me. I have never been a very patient man.

In the first week of February, six weeks before the due date, I took Prissy to her weekly doctor's visit, where they informed her that she had to have the baby induced that night. There was just too much risk with how high her blood pressure was.

They would call an ambulance from John's Hopkins in Baltimore to pick her up, as they had the best NICU in the area.

I drove home, leaving her at the hospital, and loaded up everything we had packed for the delivery.

It started snowing as I drove back to stay with Prissy until the ambulance arrived. Over the next five hours, the snow storm intensified into a full-blown blizzard. There was already 6 inches of snow on the ground, with much more expected through the night. The ambulance took a long time to get to the hospital we were waiting in, and when they arrived, they loaded up Prissy.

I told her I would be right behind her, all the way there.

As we pulled out of the parking lot, the ambulance, having four-wheel drive, and much more weight than me, quickly pulled ahead. I said a quick prayer and drove my jeep as fast as I could the normally one-and-a-half-hour drive to Baltimore.

The snow was coming down so hard I couldn't see five feet in front of the jeep. The ambulance was quickly out of sight, and I struggled to stay on the road.

I could only go about 20 to 30 miles an hour, and I spun out on the road four different times. Luckily, there wasn't anyone else on the roads.

My last spin out was on the interstate leading into Baltimore. I could almost feel God's hand pressing down on the jeep, keeping me upright. I thanked Him when my jeep came to a stop, facing the opposite direction into oncoming traffic, but I was ok.

It took me over three hours to get to the hospital, and when I finally arrived, I was one of the last people they let in the doors.

The National Guard had closed off the area hospitals because of the blizzard, and we wouldn't leave there for almost two weeks.

The much more experienced doctors and nurses at John's Hopkins told us that they would start Prissy on medicines that would keep her blood pressure down, and they wanted her to stay pregnant a little bit longer. The longer we could give Isabella to grow in her womb, the better her chances of not having complications after birth.

So, we waited. We waited for almost a week. Nerves on edge, trying to be our own advocates, we daily asked for the inducement to start.

Prissy was feeling weak, and I know I wasn't doing a good job of staying calm.

Finally, on February 9th, they deemed it too risky for Prissy to stay pregnant, and they started the inducement medicine.

They moved us into a delivery room, and it took 24 hours of torture for Prissy to finally deliver our little Isabella. The day before, another blizzard had started, blanketing the area with another foot of snow.

So, we drove to the hospital during one blizzard, and Isabella was born during another. I remember walking by the big bay windows in the hallway and looking out into a courtyard that was the original entrance to the old hospital. The snow was piled up five feet or more, and I marveled at the beauty of both the world, and the new little girl Prissy had brought into the world.

Isabella Marie, my first daughter, was born on February 10th. She only weighted a little over four pounds.

She was so small. She was half Graham's size at birth. I was amazed at how little she was, and how loud she could cry.

They rushed her to the NICU as soon as the cord was cut. Prissy didn't get the chance to hold her, and I wouldn't get the chance for a couple more hours.

The medical staff in the Neonatal Intensive Care Unit were the best in the country at what they did. They were the reason why we braved driving through a blizzard to get there. They did every test they could on little Isabella in the first hours of her life.

After everything came back satisfactory, they let me feed her. She ate like a little champ.

My little fighter was perfect. She was almost 5 weeks early, and so small, but she was perfect. God blessed me with such a precious little girl.

For the first time since I was a child, I found myself overcome with happiness to the point that I cried. I have never cried at any of my children's birth except Isabella's.

Everything we had been through to get her here made it all worth it.

She did have one thing out of the ordinary. She had a very large, what's called an "Angel's kiss" on her right side. The doctors said it would fade and eventually disappear with time, but I knew, knew in my heart, that that was a sign from God that Isabella was a real gift. I saw it as God's signature on his perfect little creation. Isabella was beautiful and perfect, and worth everything we had to go through to get her there.

Taking her back into the room where her mother was recovering, Prissy finally had a chance to hold her. I know she loved little Isabella, but she quickly gave her back to me.

I couldn't put my daughter down. I knew, no matter what, I would do anything for this little girl. She was my perfectly beautiful little daughter, and I learned very quickly that the bond between a father and his daughter is a wonderful thing.

It made me much gentler. Having a daughter took away all of my idiotic ideologies about masculinity and feminism.

This little girl could do absolutely anything she wanted to do, and she would do it better than anyone.

I would see, years later, that she would live up to that idea like the true warrior she has always been.

Chapter 20

We had been told we would be released the next day to take our new little girl home. She was eating and pooping well, and the concerns that they thought she would have, just didn't materialize. She was still perfectly healthy for being so small.

I knew that I would have to go straight to Baby's R Us, to buy every preemie outfit they had, as well as a couple of boxes of preemie diapers.

I know without a shadow of a doubt that little girl will change the world. God has been watching out for her from the very beginning.

We would eventually have some difficulties stemming from her being a preemie, and some emotional developmental problems with her, but I know in my heart she will do many great things.

She would later show us an intelligence far beyond her years, and an innate knowledge of the world and concepts she shouldn't know at a very young age.

She has her mother's drive, intelligence, and beauty. She has my stubbornness, imagination, and strength. She would overcome her challenges with grit and determination and would show fortitude and character when bad things would happen.

Later in her life, I would have to spank her one time, for a very serious infraction. She turned around, being so little still, and hit me back.

I couldn't even get mad. This little girl was so strong-willed and so strong-minded, I couldn't do anything to break that in her.

Prissy would later say I was tougher on Isabella then I was on my other children, and I didn't see it, but when I wondered why that was, it is because I have such high expectations for her.

She was a miracle when she came into this world, and God has great things in store for her.

All my children are possessed with amazing intelligence, and fortitude.

My children are all so strong. They will all succeed and do amazing things. Every one of them deserve their own chapter in this book, to describe their uniqueness and strength. Their drive and commitment to excellence. All of my children are excelling at this thing called life, and that's probably going to turn into my biggest blessing from God.

But Isabella has something special, that I pray we can foster and help develop into her meeting the potential that God gave her from birth.

I'm amazingly proud of all my children and will take time at the close of this book to explain where they all are and what they are doing, but I wanted to take this time for Isabella to know that she is an amazingly wonderful little girl, and the world is hers for the taking.

When I took mommy and baby girl home for the first time, the sky was clear. It was cold, and there was still so much snow on the ground.

We bundled Isabella up, so she was warm and sleeping, and Prissy was doing much better since the delivery. She was very tired but would have six months to get her equilibrium back. I took the girls home to rest while I went and bought out the store of every female preemie outfit they had.

I walked back into the condo to Prissy sleeping on the couch, covered in her favorite sheep blanket, and Isabella in her little rocker, sleeping next to her mother.

Prissy had put on some soft music for Isabella and lit two honeysuckle candles she had bought for us.

My heart almost burst seeing my two girls that way. They didn't know it, but in that moment, I put the bags down, got on my knees and thanked God for everything He had brought us through.

At that moment, I knew what Psalms 23 meant when it described my cup overflowing.

I still had not heard from the boys for over a year and a half, but I had a family again, and would be a father again.

My favorite job was being a father. It's very difficult at times, but it would get me though the next nine years when things weren't always so good.

But in that moment, in that warm apartment, on my knees in prayer, I looked over at my beautiful, dark haired girls, and felt joy. Real joy.

They were so beautiful, looking at them brought a song to my mind. "Leaning on the Everlasting Arms."

"How marvelous, how wonderful, is my Savior's love for me?"

Chapter 21

When Isabella was born I was 30 years old. I have left out so much that happened. I didn't talk about my short MMA fighting career.

I didn't speak about trying to start going back to college, which failed after a couple of months.

I didn't talk about the hassle of moving out of my apartment with Vicky because Prissy was uncomfortable dating me if I was living with a woman. That was in the first week of us dating.

I haven't spoken about how Prissy systemically made me get rid of almost every person in my life except her, and now my daughter.

These things were very important in my life, but not important to the main narrative. Let me say that as I cover what happened in my relationship with Prissy, it started out with the best of intentions. I thought I loved her, and didn't see, or ignored, all the red flags, early on.

I exerted my will three times in breaking up with her but came back each time. I wanted my family.

I have no ill will towards Prissy now. I just hated who I became after 10 years with her.

By my 39th birthday, I would be a completely different, almost unrecognizable person, from who I was at my 30th birthday. I became a shadow of myself.

I mentioned those other activities I did, like fighting MMA, to show you that I was an almost whole person when I met Prissy.

I was lonely, but I was filled with the Holy Spirit and had many friends and hobbies. I was surrounded with acceptance and faith. Although many in the group, including my brother, did not have a relationship with Christ, I was not judged for my faith, and in fact, was encouraged by many who asked for prayer.

I learned early in my relationship with Prissy, that while she was a spiritual person, she was not a Christian. We would visit one church two times in our 10 years together, and she judged it both times to the point that I didn't push going to church anymore.

I wanted to raise my children in the church, but Prissy didn't think that was important. So, I was made to think it wasn't important.

I would give up my will so many times in the years to come, all in the spirit of peace, and to keep my children. She knew how I felt about the boys, and she would use threats of leaving me, taking the kids, and never letting me see them again to get her way, time after time.

She was smart enough to know just how to twist my mind into doing what she wanted, and I was so tired, drugged, and beat down by the time I left her, I hardly knew who I was.

Having little Isabella at home now, and Prissy being on maternity leave, things started to calm down a little. We got into a routine. A routine that would last for the next nine years.

We were living in Waldorf, MD, in a one-bedroom condo that was nice but wouldn't work for very much longer. We had a lease until July, so we settled in to wait it out and see where we would end up after that.

Prissy's job would allow her to have an office at any Navy base in her district. Since I worked at Pax River, we thought it would make sense to move back down to deep southern Maryland, so we could both be close to daycares and work.

It would be nice to not have to drive an hour back and forth every day for work.

We settled in as new parents.

We doted on little Isabella. She was so precious, and didn't fuss much, unless we took her out.

We learned very early on that she did not like change to her environment very much. If we took her to a restaurant, or to the store, she would scream her little head off unless she was sleeping.

So, we tried to take her out during her naps.

At the time, we didn't think anything of this. Some babies are temperamental, and when we brought it up to her pediatrician, she didn't think it was out of the norm. It wasn't until Isabella was two years old that we found out that there was a problem.

As I was working long hours, and my shift changed every three months, all the rest of my free time was taken up by my family.

I didn't have time to go to the gym anymore, an activity that really had kept me grounded and in good shape for many years.

I started putting on weight.

Not a lot at first, but it got to be very noticeable over time.

It was at this time that Priscilla started a systematic culling of my friends and family. Every holiday had to be spent with her parents and siblings.

I didn't go up to Boston to see my mother's family the entire time Prissy and I were together. She had a reason for me to burn the bridges with every single one of my friends, and I went along with it.

I was happy to come home to my girls every night and cook and take care of them both. I was getting up at night with Isabella, and I noticed that at first, Prissy would help, but by the time she went back to work, I was the only one getting up at night.

She would blame sleeping too deeply to hear the baby, but I knew it was because she knew I would do it without complaint.

Priscilla's parents, Barb, and Tim, were amazing people. They had been married over 40 years, and while their health was deteriorating, I still enjoyed seeing them. We would travel into DC to see them just about every weekend. They only had one other granddaughter, who at the time, lived in Mississippi.

So, Isabella was the only grandchild they got to dote on all the time.

I spent a lot of weekends fixing up their townhouse. I replaced the downstairs flooring, painted their upstairs rooms, and re-tiled their kitchen. Their townhouse was in total disrepair, but we did what we could on the weekends that we visited.

Prissy's mother, Barb, had had a tough life. So, she was an alcoholic, and spent many weeks not getting out of bed. She smoked at least a pack of cigarettes a day and had had congestive heart failure a few years prior to me meeting her.

Prissy's father, Tim, was a great guy. I felt like he was just always in the background, taking care of Barb, and doing what she wanted.

He would start drinking beer at 7 am on the weekends and finish a 30 pack before the weekend was over. I have never seen someone drink so much beer. He would stay in the kitchen, putting around, taking a couple of hours to make breakfast, and afterwards, would move into making an early dinner.

He didn't say much. He was just there.

I came to realize that this was the kind of man that Prissy wanted. She wanted a man without an opinion, who didn't fight her domination of the house, and just handled things, quietly, and without being told to.

She slowly turned me into her father. The only solace I had was when Tim and I would go to Washington National's baseball games.

I had never liked baseball much. I thought that it was boring and didn't really understand the game.

But as Tim and I went to games, and I started watching them on television, I came to love the game, and the Nationals in particular.

We took many trips to Nationals Park every year, and even when we didn't go to the games, I would call him, and we would talk baseball in the evenings during the games.

Tim became a great father figure for me at a time that I really needed it. We would sit in section 215 of Nat's Park and talk about his time as a young boy going to the old park where the Senator's played. He saw all the greats. Jackie Robinson was his favorite.

When Jackie Robinson came to town, it basically shut down as everyone in those days went to the ballpark or sat around the radio and listened to the broadcast.

He would tell me about how the stands were segregated, and how the race wars started in DC. He was a trove of Washington DC history, and I came to find out that his family had been very influential in the city. His grandmother was the secretary to five Patent Officers. His sister was in the Secret Service. His great grandfather was the man who drove the first trolley over the Anacostia Bridge, when it opened.

And further back his family went, to being one of the original families in the area. I thought it was amazing that my children would be a part of this great family legacy. Prissy would get a book about her father's family, and even she was shocked at the family history.

Dad and I became very close. I would take him to the baseball games up until he could barely walk anymore. By that time, Prissy's parents would move in with us, and Dad would get sick and not make it.

He had been one of the strongest men I knew.

He was like my uncle, back in Texas, but much quieter. His sense of humor was drier, but his morals and convictions were the same.

I came to realize that when he was younger, and being the youngest brother of three sisters, all of which were strong personalities, he would learn to just shrug things off, and would appear placid, but I knew he was a man of very strong character and integrity.

He still held dear the reminders of his early days in his fraternity and his college days. He had collected beer steins from all over the world, and he was loved by everyone who worked for him at his job as an accountant.

I learned that his real strength was doing the hard stuff for a difficult woman. I always thought that Prissy's mother abused him, but he would just shrug it off like so many other things, and kept plodding on, drinking his beer, and giving quiet, easy advice to anyone who asked.

He would pass away in the hospital in 2014, and Mom would follow a year later, two days before Christmas.

At the time of both of their deaths, they lived with us, and I know it hit everyone hard.

It hit me very hard as well. I came to know both Prissy's parents very well. They took me in and loved me and loved my children.

The year that Mom lived with us after Dad died, she took on a new lease on life. It didn't help her in the end, but I feel like she was happy when she passed.

It was all very difficult for Prissy, but she never showed it. She grieved, but she moved on. She was a lot more like her Dad then she thought. I loved her in those times as much as she would let me, but it was very hard, and she didn't let me in.

She just squared her shoulders and kept herself to herself by her pride and fragile strength. I tried so many times to be there for her, but her and I were so much different, in our cores, that we never could understand how and what the other needed.

After Isabella was born, we eventually, moved back down to Southern Maryland, into a townhouse which we lived in for a year and a half.

When Prissy became pregnant a second time, we decided it was time to buy a house. By this time, I had lost all contact with my friends and family.

I was even forced to not talk to my brother. Prissy always had so many good reasons why I needed to erase people from my life. She made it all sound so reasonable, and for my own good.

I really believe that she thought she was doing it all for a good reason. She never had a problem moving on from people who didn't fit her agenda, and she would never look back again. I have never in my life knew anyone so cold.

I would see just how cold she could be as she persuaded me to seek out mental health services from the Veteran's Administration.

I begrudgingly went to a mental health appointment she set up for me, and as the next seven years would prove, I let them turn me into a quiet, unassuming, no opinions robot, with a mixture of strong psychotropic medication, and many sessions of therapy.

Prissy would talk to my mental health doctor, and he would increase the medicine. They diagnosed me as being bi-polar type 2, hypomanic.

The medicine they put me on, I would later learn, was unwarranted, and unneeded, but would turn me into the quiet robot that Prissy desired.

She had a way of making me feel horrible for ever having an exuberant expression of joy, or to kid around with the children, or buy myself a coffee that she didn't approve of.

She would constantly tell me I was being manic, and I had to take more medicine, or she would leave me and take the kids.

They increased my medicine to such a high level that I started losing days. I could still work, and function, but I quickly learned to live in a fugue state.

My friends at work could tell every time I would skip my pills in the morning. I was open, and funny, and easy going.

But when I took all that medicine, I was not myself at all. I went through that for seven years, until I couldn't take it anymore. I was so tired of thinking that I was going crazy.

She used the term "manic" so much, I started seeing it as my identity.

As my second daughter, Olivia Elizabeth, was born, and we had moved into our new, spacious house, a different routine set in.

I was still gaining weight, and I hated looking at myself in the mirror. I would try to steal moments of happiness with the kids while Prissy was working.

Isabella and I would laugh and play, and wrestle during the hour or so between me picking up the girls from school and Prissy getting home from work.

We would turn on music while I cooked dinner, and dance together, and laugh and joke.

As Olivia got older, we would have so much fun in that short hour to hour and a half every day.

It was our time to let our hair down and just laugh and play. But when Prissy got home, we had to be serious. We couldn't be loud, or boisterous, or I was being manic, and the kids were going along with it.

As Prissy would change into comfortable clothes, and I cooked dinner, the music would get turned down, Isabella would do her homework, and Olivia would sit in the kitchen and ask me a million questions.

This became our everyday routine.

I would live for that short time that the kids got to be kids.

I paint a bleak picture, and it wasn't always that bad, but it was a total change of environment when Prissy would get home.

But there were good times with Prissy as well.

We became a family of traditions. I have the same pictures of the kids through the years doing the same things, just being a year older in each of them.

Holidays were filled up with activities, and the kids led a rich life. Prissy made sure that they had everything she didn't have growing up.

One thing we did, at least two or three times a week was our dancing game.

While Isabella was doing homework, or the girls were watching cartoons, Prissy would come into the kitchen and yell at them that she was dancing with Daddy.

She would start dancing with me as the two girls ran in and tried to separate us. One of the girls would push Prissy out into the dining room while the other took her place dancing with me. Then the other girl would run in, ahead of her mother, and dance with me as well. Prissy would then grab one or both girls and carry them out into the dining or living room and run back in and start dancing with me again. This would go on, over and over for a couple of more minutes. It became my favorite thing we did as a family.

Looking back now, those times we would laugh and have fun with the dancing game became the thing I would think of when I thought of loving Priscilla.

I liked to think that during that game, I was seeing the real her.

Stealing quick thoughts like that kept me going through all the hard times during those years.

I'm again sitting in a coffee shop writing this, thousands of miles away from the girls and more than a year from separating from Priscilla.

Tears are streaming down my cheeks thinking of those little girls pushing their mother out of the way to dance with me. I would think back to things that I had done with the boys that were similar, and there is a pain is in my heart right now that I can't fix.

I yearn for my children today.

Right now, I have the beginnings of everything I could ever want in both purpose and drive, but without my children, I am lost and hurting.

It is late summer, 2019, and I haven't seen any of my children for almost a year.

All I have right now are these memories, and I hurt so badly from them.

I made the decisions I felt were best for everyone, but I second guess them every day.

I pray to God almost hourly to bring my family back to me. I am praying for a miracle once again in my life.

My relationship with my Lord has never been stronger, but I feel selfish most of the time because I'm not asking Him for His will, rather, I'm asking him for the miracle it would take to have my children back. All of them.

I'm in both the best place of my life, and the worse, all at the same time.

Looking back on those years I had with the girls, I feel so much pain and remorse for leaving them. I had to get away from Priscilla and her control of my life. I had to get away from the man I became because I couldn't look at him in the mirror any more.

I took on a level of self-loathing that was beyond unhealthy. Every time I tried to exert my opinion or put my foot down about something I cared about, Prissy would turn it against me and make me feel like I was crazy for ever going against her.

I had to get as far away from her as I could, and doing that, I have lost a year of my children's lives.

I made a selfish, although healthy decision, and I hate myself for it, most days. All I can do is put my hope in God to change my life, once again, to have my children back, again.

I can't live without them, and except for the peace that God gives me every time I ask for it, I'm in agony over being away from my children.

Chapter 22

In October 2012, my second daughter, Olivia Elizabeth, was born in Southern Maryland. It was a beautiful day, and as I remember back to that day, all I can recall is that everything was just easy and perfect. Prissy did not have a hard pregnancy with Olivia. And, compared to Isabella's birth, it was extremely easy on everyone.

Prissy's parents came down and stayed with Isabella for the three days that we were in the hospital with Olivia.

Prissy's mother, Barb, did not understand why I wanted to stay the entire time in the hospital with Prissy, as her husband, Tim, had not stayed with her when she had had her children. But the last time that happened was more than 30 years before, and things were just different now.

Priscilla went into labor normally with Olivia. We went to the hospital the morning of the 10th, and she was born that afternoon.

Again, compared to our first daughter's birth, Olivia was just perfect. And she was a big baby. She was perfectly healthy, cried and ate and went to the bathroom just as she was supposed to.

There were no complications, and it was an extremely festive atmosphere in the delivery room. I remember that there were three or four other mothers giving birth around us, and as we could hear them all, Prissy and I just smiled to each other that this time around, it was going to just be relaxed and easy.

Prissy was ecstatic and beautiful. There wasn't any stress, and everyone was happy. The extreme difference between the last birth we endured, and this one, was jarring. And all I could think was that God truly was blessing us with this whole experience.

I don't think any of us could handle another birth like Isabella's, and God, being all wise, gave us this extreme blessing.

Olivia was this perfect little pink ball of beautiful.

From the moment she was born, and probably for a couple of months before she was born, I have called her my Olive Bear.

Her eyes were open immediately and she took her time looking around at everyone and everything. She stopped crying very early on, earlier than all of my other children.

I could see her spirit in her eyes very early on. If Olivia has shown me anything in the last 6 years of her life, it's that she has a spirit and a heart bigger than anyone else I have ever known. She radiates love and acceptance.

That is her biggest gift, and a gift for us all.

She gets along with everyone who knows her and has many friends. Things just seem to go really easy for Olivia. I don't think that she lets on when she is hurt or having a bad day. She is always positive and optimistic. I love that about her almost more than anything. And she has been that way since she was a very small baby.

As I looked at her in her little crib in the hospital, I knew that she would always make me proud, and that I wouldn't have to worry as much about her as my other children.

Olivia is one of those people who you can tell are happy to just be alive. She has a tendency to always cheer me up. I don't even think she can help it.

There was only one scary moment in the hospital with Olivia.

During the first night we were in the room after Olivia's birth, I was forced to save her life. It's another way I know that God has looked out for all of my children.

The room was quiet, the baby was sleeping. Prissy and I had talked into the night and had finally fallen asleep around midnight. She got up at about 3am to use the bathroom. I didn't stir, until I heard a loud, male voice yelling at me to wake up and look at the baby.

I jerked violently awake, looking around, but no one was there. I looked over at Olivia, laying on her back in the transportable crib they put babies in at the hospital.

As I watched her chest rise and fall, suddenly a great gush of fluid came out of her mouth and covered her entire face. I rushed over to her as she struggled to breath.

There had been no noise at all, but she couldn't breathe. I lifted her out of the crib, turned her over, and my infant CPR training kicked in.

I held her against my forearm as I tapped her between the shoulder blades, and at the same time, I wiped the fluid from her face and out of her little nose and mouth until I heard her take a gasping breath.

She started to wail.

Her cry broke my heart, but at the same time, it was the most beautiful sound I had ever heard.

I knew at that moment an angel, or God himself woke me up in time to save Olivia's life. If I hadn't woken up, she would have choked to death on the fluid she threw up.

Prissy still hadn't heard anything and came out of the bathroom about 5 minutes later. She saw my stricken face, holding the finally calmed baby, and asked why I was shaking.

She then asked me what happened a second time, when I didn't answer. I told her the whole story.

We called a nurse in to check to make sure Olivia's airways were clear, and nothing had gotten into her lungs. Luckily, I had gotten to her fast enough that nothing got in her fragile lungs and she didn't get sick.

Today, whenever anyone asks me about my daughters, I always say the same thing. I don't know if I'm correct in saying this, but it just makes sense to me deep down.

When I speak of Isabella, I always say that Isabella will change the world. In one way or another, she will change the world. But Isabella is very chaotic in her emotions and very intense.

When I speak of Olivia, I tell people that she will save people. She may be a teacher or just a mother, but she will save people. She has a heart big enough for everyone.

It's not that my children don't have hearts, it's just that Olivia's is so big. She truly loves everyone around her and takes care of everyone. She is a true empath. She always seems to know when I'm down, and just gives me kisses and hugs and it cheers me up, every single time.

Thinking back since her birth, I can't think of one single time that I've had to discipline Olivia more than just getting on to her a little. She is an amazing little girl, and I whole-heartedly believe that she will be an amazing adult.

Olivia will be the type of adult to keep everyone together.

When this life gets hectic and chaotic, she will be the one that we all go to her house for the holidays and she will have everything prepared just the way she wants. I also believe that when I am too old to take care of myself, Olivia will be the one to make sure that I am taken care of.

One of my favorite memories about Olivia is during the times, right after I picked up the kids from school after care, we would go home, put on some music, and start dinner.

Without fail, Olivia would ask me to sit her on the counter next to where I was cooking, and she would watch me cook, and tell me all about her day, and ask me a million questions.

Sometimes this would annoy me, because I just wanted to get dinner finished, but looking back now, I cherish those memories. I see her, in her cute girly socks, her little jeans and a tank top on, because, like their mother, the first thing my daughters do when they get home is change into comfy clothes, usually just a tank top and pants.

It's the cutest thing about my girls.

But she would be sitting there, her curly brown hair usually in a ponytail or two, and she would ask me just about everything a child asks their parent on a daily basis.

She is an amazing communicator. She is as smart as her sister, but her interests lay outside of academics. She did everything just as early as Isabella did, but Olivia always has an air about her of going easy and doing it her way.

She is extremely intelligent, all of my children are, but Olivia is a lot like me in that she is a bit of a dreamer. If any of my children were going to follow me in my passion of writing, it would be Olivia. But lately, Isabella shows a very strong aptitude for it as well.

And man, would I love to read those stories from her unique perspective.

Earlier this year, Olivia fell off the monkey bars and broke her elbow. She had to have surgery and get some metal pins installed to hold the bones together while they healed. I found out just how brave my little girl is in that time.

When I saw her for the first time after the surgery, she didn't even let on that anything was wrong. She gave me the biggest grin through the pain and my heart almost burst.

I would have been a mess and wanted all the attention for what happened to me. Olivia was just counting down the days until she could get back on those monkey bars and accomplish what she wanted to do. Get to the end on her own.

So, while I say that Olivia is all heart and spirit, that little girl is a warrior as well. That may be her biggest strength. Olivia is so damn strong. And her strength is much deeper than even mine.

I pride myself on having gotten through this rough life I've had, but my strength was forged in the fire of those experiences. I had to be tempered to harden.

Olivia was already hardened by her heart and spirit, and frankly, her courage.

I worry less about Olivia than I do any of my other children. She just isn't as fazed by things as the rest of them. I think in a lot of ways, she has the best of both me and her mother.

She has her mother's beauty and perseverance. If Priscilla is anything, she is a very determined woman.

Olivia has all of that pure stubbornness. But she has my stamina and doggedness. She's a lot like me in that what she dreams to happen, she will fight to make happen until it does.

While Priscilla is very practical in her strength, and very much a realist, Olivia has my imagination and ability to hope and dream of things most would give up thinking would come to pass.

One of the biggest differences with Olivia from my other children is the bond I have with her. As a parent, you aren't supposed to have a favorite child. And I will not say here that I do, however, I don't have the bond with the rest of the children that I have with Olivia.

And I think that bond comes from a couple of different things.

First, around the time Olivia was 3 or so, she and I came up with a little saying that we say to each other every time we talk or see each other. One of us will start off by saying, "How much do I love you?" and the other person will answer the same way every time, "Forever and ever. How much do I love you?" and the first person will answer, "Forever and ever."

I have never had anything like that with any of the other kids. And it was mostly Olivia's idea, as I put her to bed every night, to start saying that. It just happened, and I cannot pinpoint exactly when it started, but it has never failed to be spoken between her and me.

And I hope, as she gets older, and things go up and down, she will always remember those words. And believe those words with her whole heart. The other child say it now as well, and it warms my heart every single time.

The second thing that makes me realize that we have such a strong bond is that Olivia really accepts me. Completely. Unlike her mother and older sister, Olivia has not once shown a hatred or anger for me leaving when I did. Every time I see her and talk to her on the phone, it's as if I've been right there next to her every single day.

That little girl is a gift to me, a balm for my restlessness and pain.

My daughters are the best of me and their mother.

Not that all my children aren't perfect, but both girls just started out on such a good note from birth, that they are my hope in life for an easier time.

Being around both of them just does something to me. They calm me. Their deep brown eyes, determined little faces, and graceful, athletic little bodies makes me feel proud to be their father, and giving them the best of me.

And they are truly the very best of me. I think if there is anything that I have done right in this world, and it wasn't even my doing, is that all of my children got the very best of me, without the experiences that broke me.

I hope that I am there when the girls are old enough to read these words. I know a long time will happen between now and that day, but when it does, I hope that we can look back on them as a 7-year-old and a 10-year-old, and that everything I've written here has just been intensified in their lives, and that they are successful in everything that they choose to do.

I have no doubt that they will be.

I think, many years from now, both girls will be what my father was for my family when I was their age now.

They will both hold us all together.

Olivia will be the glue that makes my little family into a huge success. She is the rock of my children. All of them. And she will be my memory when I'm gone.

Isabella will be the practical, intellectual one, keeping everyone organized and goal-orientated.

I love them both so much, and I hope, as they reads these words, I am in the room for them both to come give me a big hug and ask me, "How much do I love you?"

And I can look into their beautiful faces, and their deep brown eyes that look so much like my own, and say, "Forever and ever, my babies. Forever and ever."

Chapter 23

So, how did I get here? What happened to drive me so far from my family?

It started in earnest in May of 2016. In a lot of ways, it started that day, in 2009, when I got up the courage to talk to Prissy outside of our apartment building.

After seven years together, Prissy and I decided to finally get married. We planned the day on our seventh anniversary, so we could keep the same date. By this time, her parents had come to live with us, and had both passed away.

We had spent the beginning of 2016 planning her little sister's wedding and had spent so much money on our part of that huge wedding, we decided to just go easy on ours, and have it at the court house on the day of our anniversary, which happened to be a Wednesday.

Her sister and her sister's fiancé, Colin, were the only ones there. We had invited her two other brothers, but neither came.

This was a continuing theme in her family. We supported everything they did, but they didn't come to any of my family's activities.

It really bothered Priscilla, and she would go on to not talk to her brothers much in the next couple of years.

But her sister and Colin, we hung out with and saw more, than anyone else. They became the only family that we did anything with.

It was a beautiful late spring day, May 24th, 2016, and Prissy had bought a beautiful white dress for the occasion. I was in a dark blue suit, and we had flower arrangements made for the small wedding.

The courthouse sits on a beautiful piece of property, and they routinely perform marriages outside, when it is nice.

So, we gathered under the trees in the front of the old courthouse in Leonardtown, MD, and said our vows to each other.

On that day, I overlooked the years of emotional abuse that I tried, every day, to ignore. I wanted to love this woman, and share my life with her, and raise our girls together.

I lived for the few moments of happiness in an otherwise dismal life with her. Even on this day, it went exactly how she wanted it, and she practically wrote my vows for me.

As we drove to our favorite restaurant for a small lunch with the girls and Prissy's sister and Colin, I thought back to the day I proposed and gave her the engagement ring I had bought, and I started to regret what I had just done on that courthouse lawn on this crisp, late spring day.

I had had the whole weekend planned to propose to her. I planned with Prissy's brother and his girlfriend, who both worked for Marriot in downtown Washington DC.

I reserved a room, and they would spread rose petals on the bed, and have wine and chocolate waiting for us.

I planned with Colin, who was working on his Master of Music at a prestigious college in Baltimore to have a couple of his fellow students who played stringed instruments to be playing along the river near the mall in DC.

I was going to take Prissy to DC and take her for a walk, stopping by the music playing students, and unbeknownst to her, would propose with our favorite classical song, Pachelbel's Canon, playing.

I had it all planned out, and when I told her to plan a weekend away, she kyboshed the whole deal. She said we couldn't afford a trip to DC, no matter what I was doing.

So, I had sprung into Plan B. I asked her what she would allow, and she begrudged agreed to a hotel in nearby Solomon's Island, and a dinner in DC.

As the weekend came closer, I made a new plan. I would take her to the beach where we had our first kiss, at Greenwell State Park, and propose there, and then take her to a nice dinner in DC, and back to the hotel for the weekend.

As the day drew near that we could get away for our first weekend away from the kids in more than 3 years, her sister and Colin came to babysit. We loaded our bags in the car, and I started driving towards Greenwell.

I had a letter written to her in my pocket, and I was planning to read the love letter, get on one knee, and give her the ring that she had picked out.

As we drove towards the park, she knew what I was going to do. She asked,

"You aren't taking me to that beach to propose, are you? Because I really don't want that."

"Well I'm not now." I said. I was crushed.

So, the only thing I could think to do on such short notice, and now having to change the plan again, is to drive out on Solomon's Island and park by the water and propose that way.

When we got to the parking spot overlooking Patuxent River, there were people in cars around us. I wanted to get out into the overcast afternoon and propose at least with the smell of the water and feeling the spray of it hitting the rocks as a backdrop for some kind of romance. She didn't want to get out of the car, or for other people to see us.

So, I sat in the car, reading her the love letter I had written to her, expressing my undying love and commitment, and espousing her virtues. I took out the ring, and as I was unable to get on my knee to propose, just gave it to her in the box. I was beyond upset.

She had ruined my proposal twice. She kept saying that apparently, I didn't know her well enough to do it to her liking. I should have taken that ring and threw it in the river. I guess I never really did know her.

We ended up going to a restaurant in Annapolis, as she didn't want to be too far away from the girls. After dinner, we drove back to the hotel in silence, and did not make love that night, like I had planned.

It was the worst possible marriage proposal I could have made, and I felt like I had no choice. Every plan, every kind of romance I tried to bring into it, was against what she wanted.

I was made to feel like I didn't even try because I didn't do it how she would want it done.

To this day, I can't think of any other way to do it. I could never find out exactly what she wanted, every single day.

I was a failure at our relationship, our eventual marriage, and she made me feel like I never knew her. I have no idea how to make that woman happy.

I would later understand that she was not a naturally happy person to begin with, so nothing I could do would change that for her. I tried every day, in small ways and large to try to make her happy, and it never worked.

I'll give you an example.

181

Every evening, after we got the kids to bed, and Prissy had her shower, we would have our alone time.

What this meant, is that we would have a cocktail or tea, and watch CNN.

I hated CNN with a passion. I did not agree with anything they said, or the opinions they had. But Prissy loved it. She would start arguments with me because I grew up in a conservative environment, and she was a liberal.

The arguments would turn ugly, and she wouldn't talk to me for a couple of days. This happened a couple of times a week.

All I wanted to do was watch baseball, but since her father died, there was really no reason in her eyes why I needed to watch the Nationals every night.

While we were watching CNN, she would always expect me to rub her shoulders or feet. I never really minded doing this, except the nights that my hands hurt.

I worked as an aircraft mechanic, and often had to work in small, uncomfortable places, doing intricate work that would make my hands cramp. I developed arthritis in both hands, so it was sometimes extremely painful to rub her shoulders or her feet at night.

She would get so upset with me if I didn't massage her but would get even more upset if I told her I could do it for a little while until I couldn't handle the pain anymore. She would yell at me that she would rather not have any kind of massage if I were just going to do it, "half-ass."

She would make me feel so bad that I didn't rub her feet or shoulders when my hands and back were cramping. I felt like a failure.

After a couple of years of this, I started thinking the same thoughts every time I massaged her. What did she do for me?

I racked my brain wondering what she did for me. During the few and far between times we would have sex, it was always to get her to orgasm, and I would take care of myself. She would be the most amorous when she wanted to be pregnant. But otherwise, I think she did it out of duty.

She had told me from week one that she wanted three kids. No more, no less.

Every time she felt it was time to have another child, she would seduce me, and do what she could for me to orgasm inside of her.

I built up a wall, not allowing me to orgasm inside a woman for years after this. But I would ask myself, what did she do for me?

The one time I posed this question to her, she told me that she did everything for me, every day.

She would go grocery shopping and get me my favorite candy.

She would throw away my old underwear and buy me new.

She told me she went without her expensive makeup and perfume now for me.

She didn't say that she had to have the kids in the most expensive private school in southern Maryland, and our daycare bill was sometimes twice what our mortgage was.

I looked down at myself, weighing over 280 pounds at this time, and hated the way my body looked in the mirror.

Did she let me go to the gym? No. She would say she liked me with the Dad Body, and we couldn't afford a gym membership anyway, and I didn't have time for it as well.

I would look at this woman that I married, and ask, every single day, what did she do for me?

We didn't go to church like I wanted. We weren't active and were getting so badly out of shape.

We didn't eat well. We made sure to always have the four food groups on the table, and the kids had fruit and veggies every night.

But we ate horribly.

It got to be, in the end, that the only good things in my life were my children.

I learned to hate Prissy.

It was my fault that I allowed it to get this bad, but I felt like I couldn't fight her anymore. I remembered back to those early days when I would have fire and opinions and didn't let her walk all over me. Where did that guy go?

Now, I was a fat, out of shape, depressed man, who only lived for his children and hated his wife and his job. I had to make some changes.

Right after we got married, I decided to go back to school.

I didn't have much more left, and I investigated different majors.

After Prissy and I researched it, we found that getting a degree in Communications would help me get off the flight line.

So, I enrolled in the college she graduated from, and spent the next two years doing classes every single night.

The kids would urge me on, and for once, Prissy was supportive in something. She always hated the fact that I didn't have my degree. I knew she wanted the best for me, but I felt in a way, it reflected on her as well.

So, I would brew a pot of coffee, and after giving the kids their baths, I would get on my computer and do my classes.

I loved every minute of it. I loved writing papers again. I loved putting my headphones on and listen to music while I worked.

Just like I'm doing right now, I have my headphones on, and I'm listening to Christian music while writing this.

I enjoyed the challenge of school so much.

In 2018, I decided to use my almost-completed education and my experience of so many years working on airplanes to apply for jobs doing Technical Writing.

Almost immediately I was interviewed for a tech writing job on the new Navy Triton platform.

I gleefully and happily resigned my position working on the flight line and vowed to never go back.

I bought some dress clothes, and went to work for a new contracting company, writing maintenance manuals for the new Triton.

I learned how to write code and loved every minute of the new job. I was working in an office and dressing up for work every day.

I got a higher security clearance and made more money than I had previously. I absolutely loved working at a desk every day.

My overall demeanor changed. And I started seeing my value.

After so many years of being less than Prissy in the professional world, I finally felt on equal footing.

I was doing something that used my mind, and not my body.

I started feeling happy again.

I also started contacting my brother, who lived in Florida, again. I had to do it from my work phone, as Prissy checked my cellphone every night.

I told him that my company was flying me down for a week-long training in Jacksonville every month for three months.

I asked him if he would drive up to see me while I was there. I hadn't seen him in almost seven years. I missed him miserably.

Another thing happened right before this time to change my life a little more. Prissy became pregnant with our third child.

This was going to be my sixth child, and I had been telling Prissy for a couple of years that I wanted to get a vasectomy. She would not allow it until we had three children together.

So, when she became pregnant for the third time, I made an appointment with my urologist for a vasectomy. When Prissy found out about it, she made me cancel it. She wanted to make sure this baby was healthy and then she would think about letting me get snipped.

My fourth son, Alexander Lloyd, was born in April 2017. He was born on opening day for the Nationals, and as Prissy was in labor, I was able to watch the opening ceremony and the first game of the season, in which my favorite player, Bryce Harper hit a home run.

I felt that home run was for my new son.

When Alex was born, we gave him a baseball pacifier. The hospital staff were all aware of Alex's auspicious start to life.

I was a proud, proud father.

The labor and delivery went well, and Alex was a perfectly healthy baby boy. There were no issues, and Prissy was up walking that day.

Now, we had Prissy's dream of being married, owning a nice, big house, and having three healthy, beautiful, dark-haired children. We both had great jobs and two nice cars in the driveway.

I should have been so very happy, but I started feeling more and more miserable.

I was living Prissy's dream.

I fit the mold she had in her goals of the quiet, unobtrusive husband, without an opinion, who was there to just plod around the kitchen, getting fat, and drinking beer. I didn't drink a lot of beer, but I barbequed on the weekends, mowed the lawn, took out the trash, gave the kids' baths every night, and tucked them all in to bed.

I woke up at night with the babies and I worked a job I enjoyed now, but that was still limiting me. I knew Prissy was fulfilled at this time. She had her happy family she could be proud of, but I was miserable every single day.

I started to rebel. I started to get my fire back. I stopped taking the medicine and felt better for the first time in years. By Christmas, 2017, I knew that I had to start working on an escape plan.

It killed me thinking about the kids growing up with divorced parents, but it was better than the fighting we did, and the misery I felt every day.

I didn't want to run away from the kids again and vowed I would do everything I could to stay in their lives. Alex was so small, but I felt in my soul I had to get away from Prissy. I had to change my life for me, and to get myself back.

I had to find myself, and I had to make drastic changes to find who I really was again.

The first time my company flew me down to Florida, and I saw my brother for the first time in seven years, it was decided in my mind.

Jasper would go on to help me get away from Prissy, and I would go through an eventual year of so many ups and downs it was as if anything that had happened in my life before this didn't matter a bit. I still had a fire to get through, and God has a way of giving us exactly what we need. What I needed, was a huge wake up call.

Half of 2018, and most of 2019 would test me in ways I couldn't imagine.

If I looked ahead and saw what was in store for me during that year, I would have gladly stayed with Prissy and the kids and became comfortable in the stability of that family.

I would have remained miserable and would probably die early, but I wouldn't be tossed around emotionally and financially and physically like I did in the last year.

Because in the last year, I would find myself again.

I would find God again.

I tried to find the love of my life, but there would be a cost. A high, high cost.

I would not wish this year on anyone. And by the end of it, I would be so much stronger for it.

I AM so much stronger from it.

But first, there was one last experience I had with Prissy towards the end that would seal the fate of our marriage forever.

We had rented a new movie, a musical, and I was excited to watch it. "The Greatest Showman" would go on to become one of my favorite movies, and the soundtrack would go with me for miles and miles as I would eventually drive the roads between Florida and Maryland to see the kids every month.

After we finished the movie, before another word was spoken, Prissy said something to me that echoed one of the songs in the movie.

The song, called "A Million Dreams" talked about how the protagonist in the movie, the venerable B.T. Barnum had grown up with dreams bigger than life in his mind.

Prissy turned to me as soon as the movie was off, and in a flippant tone of voice said to me,

"When are you going to do something to turn our lives around? When are you going to give me everything you ever promised me? Where are your dreams?"

I couldn't reply. I had no words for how she made me feel. I just knew that no matter what I did in my life, it would never be good enough for her.

She never cheated on me or abandoned me. But she messed up my view of myself and my opinions and goals to an extent that I had no idea who the hell I was.

And she thought through all of that, that she was the victim in our relationship. That she had to sacrifice so much to be with me, like she had been doing me a colossal favor the entire time just by staying with me, and she was a saint for everything she did, day in and day out.

Thinking about the smug look on her face as she belittled all I had worked so hard for up until then makes me sick.

I had real dreams when we met. I had this story in me the whole time. I had the gifts that God gave me to tell stories, and to inspire those who read my words to know that there is so much happiness in the world no matter what you have gone through.

But I didn't want to soil my gifts by her opinions of every single word I would write, or every single thing I would do to find my peace and happiness once again.

I cannot imagine the amount of ego and pride in that woman's mind and body to make her think that she was the one who had to put up with me and deserved something grand and amazing for it.

The rest of this book will describe the last 14 months, and how I went from being married, living in a five-bedroom house and having complete stability, and financial freedom, to sleeping in my car in the Florida heat, in a Walmart parking lot for nights at a time, with no money, no job, and finally, finding some happiness and joy.

Blessed are we in our affliction, for the benefits and rewards God gives us in that time, and the wisdom we gain from our trials.

Chapter 24

At the start of 2018, Priscilla and I were not doing very well in our relationship.

But the kids were doing well. The girls were involved in school, social activities, soccer, swimming, and looking forward to summer camp. Isabella had a best friend that she spent every day with at school, and Olivia was learning independence at the private school we had her and Alex enrolled in.

Alex was doing well adjusting and had been walking and starting to talk. Prissy was doing well in her career, moving up to a higher management position a year before, and was making good money.

As I closed in on finishing my degree, I finally went to work for a job off the flightline. I was working in an office and loving it.

All of that was so good, and would have been enough, if Prissy and my relationship was worth anything. She would tell you she was happy in it, but I was full of contempt and bitterness.

I don't know if I was just feeling uneasy, or if my needs really weren't being met.

We fought all the time, and I started to feel like I didn't know who I was, and I didn't like who I saw in the mirror every morning.

I felt invalidated and had no say in what was happening in my life. But I also wasn't going a good job communicating or trying to make it work.

I had given up.

I was lost and felt empty again. I know Prissy felt this. I just wasn't where I wanted to be, and I didn't like who I was married to.

I felt trapped and unhappy every day. A lot of it was not Prissy's fault. I think she did the best she could with who she was. I just didn't like who she was.

I knew she was an amazing mother. The kids loved her, and she sacrificed a lot of what she wanted to make sure they had everything they wanted.

By this time, I had sued Victoria for joint custody of the boys, and they were coming out regularly to Maryland to know their siblings and see a world outside of the Texas panhandle.

I was getting to know the boys again, and I felt really blessed for that. So much time had gone by though. They didn't know me anymore, and I was trying to change that. They called me by my first name instead of "Dad" and I remembered back to how I wouldn't call my biological mother "mom."

I didn't blame them, but it stung. Prissy had spent almost a year fighting Victoria for the custody hearing. She got so involved I felt like she was doing all the fighting and not doing what I wanted in the process. It worked, but at a huge cost.

As winter turned into a warm spring, and the trees started throwing off all the pollen that hurt my allergies every year, the fighting between Prissy and I intensified.

I was so unhappy.

At work, I would look up dating sites and look at massage parlors in DC. I finally broke down and went to an Asian massage parlor for fake intimacy.

I was uneasy the whole time and felt dirty afterwards. I was not good at cheating, or hiding things from Prissy, so I accidently left a sticky note in my car with the address of the parlor. She found this and looked up what it was.

She had never trusted me, and now I didn't blame her.

So, three months before I left, I had to start sleeping on the couch downstairs, and didn't have much to do with my wife.

She was betrayed, and I did it to her. It was incredibly hard to feel bad about it though. I knew that I had made a drastic mistake, but with all the fighting about everything else, and never being happy with her, I just didn't care anymore.

As it got worse and worse, I withdrew deeper into myself. My work suffered, and the kids could feel it. They knew, instinctively that mom and dad weren't doing well.

It was May again. I had such a phobia about the month of May. On the weekend before I left, we had planned to go to Ocean City, MD for a small family vacation.

The kids had a blast, but Prissy and I argued the whole trip there and back. It just wasn't getting any better and had been bad for a lot of years.

When we got back home, I decided to leave. It may have appeared manic what I did, but I felt deep in my heart that I had to go. I had to get as far away from Prissy as I could. I had to find myself again, and try, once again, to get my life together for my own mental health.

Once again, I would be running away from my children, but again I justified it by thinking they were better off without me.

It was a Tuesday. I was working but knew that I wanted to run. I got a text message from Prissy, again, bashing me, and telling me how I messed it all up. And I did, but I wasn't alone in it.

I sent an email to my boss, packed up my work computer and some files, and headed out the door. I got home and wrote Prissy a letter.

I have no idea what it said other than telling her I was driving to Florida, and I wouldn't be coming back except to see the kids.

I packed a bag, grabbed whatever I felt I needed for the immediate future, and headed for the door.

I pulled two thousand dollars from our savings account and gassed up my car. I hit the road by mid-morning. I knew I had a couple of hours before she went home for lunch and saw the note.

It was about two hours later that she started blowing up my phone. Then her sister and her husband started blowing up my phone with calls and texts.

Everyone thought I had gone crazy.

Prissy called my sisters; she called my aunt. She did everything she could to get the people I love to tell me to turn around and go home.

I ended up turning off my phone.

As the miles stretched behind me, I felt like I could breathe again. I was deathly worried about the kids. I was ashamed, and tears fell as I thought about them, and them crying that I wasn't there that night to cook dinner and dance with them and tuck them into bed.

To this day, fourteen months later, I can't think of the girls without a lump forming in my throat, and tears coming to my eyes.

Lately, I have been doing everything I can to get them back in my life.

As I got into South Carolina, I checked my phone messages. There was a voicemail from a police officer in Maryland. He told me to stop where I was going and turn around and go to the hospital.

Prissy had called them and told them that I was having a break with reality. I was a danger to myself.

But I knew I had to do this. I had to get away. I had to find myself again.

That day, as I drove south, and the day turned into night, I started praying again for the first time in a long time. I asked God if I was doing the right thing, over and over. I cried out to Him to lead me to do the right thing.

I couldn't go back home.

Prissy had been poison to me and my mental health. I brought all my medications with me, but I didn't take them again.

From that day on, after I flushed them all down the toilet, I didn't take another psychotropic medication.

I would go through about a week of withdrawals and dizzy spells coming off them the way I did, but my mind was clear again.

I was in no way happy, but I felt clear.

The next day, as I finally drove into Florida, I felt a renewing of my mind and spirit. I asked God for peace, and He gave it to me.

I had no idea what the future held, but I felt drawn to Florida, and I felt like God wanted me there.

I got to my brother's home and he greeted me with a huge hug and a cigar and beer. I didn't even unload my car.

I sat on his porch, each of us smoking our favorite cigar, and I told him that I had no idea what I was doing, but I had to do it.

He agreed that Prissy had never been good for me. The stability and money didn't cover for the misery I felt being with her.

We were just a bad fit from the beginning. We were complete opposites, and I couldn't spend the rest of my life just being in the background, silent, and taking care of everything. I had to be more than that in a relationship.

I had to feel loved.

I knew I wasn't looking for a relationship any time soon, but the possibility was nice. I had to work on myself, in a big way. It would start the next day.

My job let me work from home for the first couple of months I was in Florida. I quickly found an apartment near my brother and worked every day.

But after two months, they rescinded the offer, and fired me. I had to cash out my 401k to live on.

I started looking for a job right away. I found one about a month later and went from being a tech writer for the Navy, to being one for the Air Force.

I moved further south to work at that job and lived in West Palm Beach.

When I moved, I finally decided I was ready to start dating. I knew that all of that was done on dating sites now, so I signed up for a few. At first, nothing really came of it, until finally it did.

I had traveled back up to Maryland a handful of times to see the kids and to get my things from the house.

Prissy and I did not talk anymore, because all she would do was still try to control everything I did. She had great advice about our impending divorce, and how I should be arranging my finances to help her as much as I could, and she threatened me every day with how much I would be paying in child support and spousal support. What she didn't consider was that I was paid very well in Maryland. I had made over 90k the year before.

But in Florida, doing the same job, I was paid less than half of that. And I was considered highly paid for Florida.

There just was a different way of living down there.

I had moved into an apartment with a roommate, a gay, black man named Joe, who became one of my closest friends. He was dating a very nice man named Elliot, and they made a very cute couple.

I know a lot of Christians will read that last sentence and think that I was allowing myself to be around sin, but they had real love, and as God is love, it's not up to me to judge their lives.

I knew that they were good men, with lots of integrity and love. They were too genuine to be cast as sinners and judged for how they were made.

I also had a couple of friends at work, and one, a man named Frank, was incredibly spiritual. He was an amazing Christian, and really inspired me to get closer and closer to God.

Which I did.

I was in such a good place, mentally and physically.

I was going to the gym, eating well, and losing a ton of weight. Money was tight, but I was making do.

The apartment we lived in sat on a golf course, and there was a lake right under our balcony. It was a beautiful setting to sit and read in the evenings.

I also started walking. There was a road around my neighborhood, surrounding the golf course, which was about 4 miles to walk. I started slow but got to where I could walk the whole circle twice in about an hour and a half. Some evenings I ran it. It really made me feel good.

Another thing I started doing, almost immediately after moving to Florida was intermittent fasting. I had to lose my weight and get back into shape. When I drove south, I weighed 305 pounds. My knees hurt every time I walked up stairs, and I had bad acid reflux.

I started losing weight at an astonishing rate. A year later, I would have lost 140 pounds, and weighted under 200 for the first time since I met Victoria.

My knees didn't hurt anymore, and since I started eating better, my acid reflux, as well as my blood pressure went down.

My self-esteem slowly came back. I also started going back to church. My faith in God was slowly restored, and I felt so strongly that God was moving me towards something great.

I had no idea what that was, but I knew that it was going to shape the rest of my life.

I was in a real transitional phase in my life. I was lonely, very lonely, but I was starting to feel better about it. I felt like I took the time to get to know myself better, and I started liking who I saw in the mirror in the mornings.

I was enjoying my job, but still felt unfulfilled sometimes. I met some friends, and still hung out with my brother at least once or twice a week. Everything seemed to be clicking well. I had a life again, but it was still very transitional, and I still felt drawn towards something God had on the horizon. I still felt that I wasn't living up to my potential, but I was getting closer every day.

The life I found in Florida was so very different than the life I had lived up until then. After my first marriage, I partied, drank, smoked weed, and slept with any woman who would let me. Lots let me.

But there in Florida, now single and doing pretty well, I didn't want to do those things anymore. And I was starting to see a little light on the horizon when it came to being alone with myself. It was tough, but I was tougher.

It took from May until November of 2018 to start feeling better about myself, and to feel like I was making progress on my mental health.

I had not taken one pill for all that time, and I felt steady and well. I knew I had been misdiagnosed by the VA, who went off my family history and the word of Prissy.

I wasn't bipolar. I did have PTSD.

And I had plans to work on that.

A lot of people have asked me how I lost all that weight.

I want to go over my process to lose the 140 pounds that I lost while in Florida. I did some studying, as I'm keen to do, and I felt like intermittent fasting would be the best way to go.

It took a month or two to get to where I was doing the actual fasting for 18 to 20 hours a day and get to the point where I was doing what is called OMAD, or one meal a day.

I was counting my calories every day and making sure I was keeping my intake under 1000 a day. After a couple of months of this, I started working in gym time 4 times a week.

I lost the weight rather quickly.

I was very proud of the progress I was making, and when I decided to start dating again, I knew I brought more to the table being in great shape, rather than being a fat tub of lard.

By the time November rolled around, I was down 80 pounds, and feeling good.

In November, I signed up for Tinder.

I did it out of curiosity at first, without real expectations of finding the love of my life on it, but what I found would rock me to the core, once again, and I learned just how broken I still was.

I healed a lot in that time, but it just took one little push to make all those old fears and betrayals come up.

I was about to learn some lessons that were painful, but also every important. Extremely important.

I was about to meet a woman I would later nickname "The Pirate."

The Pirate would show me just how much more work I needed to do on myself and would bring back every old pain to the very surface.

My journey had just started. I felt good about who and what I was, and where I was, but I was so wrong.

I was still broken.

I would soon learn just how broken I really was, physically, and more importantly, mentally.

Chapter 25

In November of 2018, I made a profile on Tinder.com.

I had been on there for about a week when I matched with a really pretty blonde woman in her mid-40s. Her pictures made her seem kooky, so I swiped right on her, and got a match.

We started chatting while I was working in my small cubicle at work, and it was a great conversation from the beginning.

She told me she was a Christian and had two teenage children. She had just gotten out of a seventeen-year marriage that was the worse time of her life. I could sympathize with that, and we just really hit it off.

She invited me out to a trivia contest that night near where I lived, but before I could solidify the date, she disappeared. Her profile just disappeared.

I was really bummed out because I thought the conversation had gone so well. I remember texting my brother and asking him if a profile disappeared, what did that mean. He told me that she had unmatched me.

I was upset but went about my day. That evening, I did consider going to the trivia contest to see if she was there, but if she had unmatched me for whatever reason, I didn't want to seem like a crazy person.

The next morning, I was perusing Tinder again, when her profile popped back up for about 1 minute. This time, I wrote down her first name, which was a weird spelling. She disappeared again.

I knew which town she lived in, and now I had her unique spelling of her name, so I did a little research. I found someone by the name in her town and did a reverse search for a phone number. I got two matches!

So, hesitantly, I texted both numbers with a basic text saying, "Hey, this is J.L. I was talking to a woman yesterday with this name and found this number. I hope this isn't too weird, but I was enjoying our conversation."

One of the numbers responded and said, "This is her, I'm so glad you found me. My Tinder is messed up and kicked me off yesterday. I got back on this morning to cancel it."

I also learned that the other number I had texted was her ex-husband's phone number. I never heard anything more about that, but thought it was funny that he got that text.

So, that's what had happened. She didn't un-match me. Tinder messed up her profile.

From that moment, we started chatting for hours. It was incredibly easy to talk to her. She was open, and smart, and accomplished. We made a date to meet at a cider distillery the next evening. I was looking forward to it quite a bit.

I got to the cider distillery earlier than our date because I wanted a little liquid courage, and to check the place out. They had a sampler of the different cider's they made, and I tried six of them.

I told the owner and the bartender that I was there for my first Tinder date. They warned me about Tinder dates, so I asked them to keep an eye on the door and let me know if I was getting catfished.

But I needn't have worried. She walked in wearing a tight blue dress, with high heels, and looking great. She greeted me with a hug and a kiss on the cheek. I asked her to sit, and she got the sampler as well. We shared the different ciders off each of our samplers, and the talk was fun and quick. She was very attractive, and I liked her from the start. It started raining outside as we sat there talking and drinking different ciders. When she got up to use the bathroom, both the owner and the bartender gave me a high five. She was extremely attractive.

After about an hour and a half she suddenly said she had to get home. I was confused by her sudden exit, but as it was my first Tinder date, I didn't think much of it.

I told her I would walk her to her car, and as it was pouring rain outside, we both got drenched. She told me to get into her car, and she would drive me to the other side of the parking lot to my car. Her air conditioning was on, and I instantly froze.

She drove me over to my Explorer, and before I got out, we had our first kiss.

It was cold, and wet, and we were both shivering. So, as far as first kisses go, it wasn't that great. I told her I would text her later, and I got out into the rain and watched her drive away. I went home and texted her goodnight.

She sent me a text saying that she was sorry she had to go suddenly, but she had started her period that night and had to get home for that.

I understood and asked if she wanted to meet again. She said, of course, and invited me to a rodeo the next night. I told her that I knew a little bit about rodeos and would see her there.

The next night, we went to the rodeo, and took our first picture together. I really liked her. She dressed in tight jeans and a country shirt. I wore tight jeans and my cowboy hat. We hit it off and decided to go on a weekend trip the next weekend.

That weekend started a whole slew of adventures together. It seemed like almost every weekend, and a couple nights a week we would go out and do stuff.

She was kind of exhausting to try to keep up with, and my budget certainly couldn't keep up.

She made quite a bit more money than me, and working from home, she always got bored. That would really come into play later.

But we were having fun. A lot of fun. And the sex was amazing. I did things with her I had never done before. She was adventurous, and outgoing, and down for anything.

We did so much experimenting with each other. I thought, very early on, that this was the woman for me. We would go to church every Sunday, and she always looked and acted proper, unless we were alone.

I found she had a very dirty mind and liked to live out fantasies. I was ok with it, because I thought she was just doing it with me and was totally as into me as I was into her.

Man was I wrong.

I learned through conversations, that since she got divorced a year and a half earlier, she had lived her life how she wanted to. She had dated a lot of men and had a lot of fun. There wasn't anything wrong with that, as she wasn't in a relationship, but with me, she wanted the relationship.

A month into our relationship, while lying in bed one lazy Sunday afternoon, she told me she had something to tell me. She told me that she had two lovers in her life that she wanted to keep having sex with, as well as have the relationship with me.

I found out that for those four weeks, she had continued having sex with these men while I was working. She worked from home and would just invite them over for her fun in the mornings, and I would see her in the evenings, never knowing what she had done.

To say that this messed with my fragile self-esteem is sugar coating it.

204

It messed me up really bad.

I told her I had to think about it. I left, and at work the next day, she started sending me podcasts and videos from people who taught that monogamy didn't work anymore.

All of this broke the fragile trust I had for her, and for women in general. I thought back to the times we went to church together and she would whisper in my car that she wanted to make love to me right there. I thought that was inappropriate but shrugged it off.

I shrugged a lot of things off with her. But I couldn't go through the cheating anymore. So, I went to her house and broke up with her. This was a week before Christmas.

I texted her the next morning and told her I thought I had made a mistake. I was starting to again feel the loneliness that I had battled for so long, and I thought we had something real going, but I hurt her feelings and she told me we should take two weeks off and talk again then.

It was a torturous two weeks. The worse day was Christmas.

A week before I broke up with the pirate, I started getting a pain between my shoulder blades. It got so bad that I went to the VA hospital and they took scans of my spine.

I had severe arthritis in my cervical spine.

This was pinching the nerves from my spinal cord and was causing numbness down my left arm. My left fingers tingled all day, and I knew this was something bad.

Over the next three weeks, my muscles in my left arm atrophied. So, the VA gave me very strong medications to try to stop the pain, but it never helped. Driving was the worse. I was in constant, foot tapping pain.

Christmas eve, I was so lonely. My brother invited me to his house to spend time with him and his girlfriend, Dannie, and her brother, Scott. It was a nice day.

We exchanged presents, made a lot of food, and it was just nice to be around people. Jasper let me spend the night but asked if I would go home Christmas day, so he could spend it with Dannie. I didn't mind but did not look forward to being in my apartment alone on Christmas.

The next day, as I was driving back to West Palm Beach, the pirate texted me Merry Christmas. I had not heard from her in a week and a half. I asked her if we could talk and she said she would call me that evening. I missed her a lot, and looking back now, I should have stayed as far away from her as I could. But I looked forward to the call.

When it didn't come, I was devastated.

Christmas day, I was in my apartment, alone, and feeling sorry for myself. I was alone in the world, and in such extreme pain. I had called the little kids in Maryland, but they were going to Prissy's family's house, and didn't have time for their absent father.

I knew it was all my fault, but that day was easily the worse of my life. And then the pirate did not call me. I drank whiskey until my back and arm didn't hurt anymore and ordered in Chinese food.

I went to bed early and wanted to cry for the first time since Isabella was born.

I was once again glancing over the lip of that hole I had found myself in one other time in my life.

The jail cell in Utah, twelve years previous.

Chapter 26

The day after Christmas, the Pirate called me and wanted to talk. So, I went to her house, and we sat on her patio and talked about where we were and what we wanted.

I found out that while we had been separated, she had slept with three guys, and had plans to go away the next weekend with a guy she had been seeing for a week.

I have no idea why I didn't just run away right then. But, as we talked, we decided that we wanted to be exclusive with each other, if we still did things she wanted to do, but we did it all together. She was still exploring her sexuality and I knew that I would have to step outside my comfort zone to please her.

From that day on, I went to her house every day, and spent every night with her for the next four months. We started making plans to go to couples' therapy, but only actually went together twice.

The therapist was a very nice older man. He wanted to see me individually, so I made plans to see him every week. She also was seeing him individually, also once a week.

He helped me overcome a lot of the pain from when my father died. He used a new technique with me called Emotional Transformation Therapy.

I became a huge proponent of the therapy and would tell anyone about it that would listen. I was able to sleep for the first time in a very long time after my second session. I cried for two days straight after the first session.

It helped me so much, and today, I am continuing therapy, with a new diagnosis.

I learned that I have a condition called C-PTSD.

It hasn't been studied as much as regular PTSD, but there is still a lot of information on it, and the diagnosis really answers a lot of questions about how I have responded to things, and why I have made decisions the way that I have in my life.

In February, after the Pirate and I had been back together for two months, I purchased tickets to a very important conference in Jacksonville. It was a conference given by the man who wrote "The Five Love Languages", Gary Chapman.

The man himself was giving the conference, and it was geared towards married couples, but dating couples, and even single people were encouraged to attend.

We decided to go to it for several reasons. First, she had attended the same conference fifteen years earlier with her husband and had horrible results. Her husband would not do the exercises with her, and showed that it wasn't important to him, but it was to her. When she was younger, and wrote papers in school, she had a thing about trying to figure out the Love Languages of the characters.

When she told me that story, I thought it would be an amazing experience for her to show that I was a man who cared, who would do all the exercises with her, and show that I was capable of real love and commitment in the relationship.

I knew the theory was important to her, and I wanted to make it a new memory for her. We were going to make a weekend getaway out of it.

We would do the conference on Saturday morning, and then spend the rest of the weekend in St. Augustine, a place I had always wanted to visit.

So, the drive up on Friday was great. We stayed at a hotel that night and made very passionate love to each other. I was very excited about the conference the next day.

When we got to the church where it was held, it started great, but went downhill very quickly. As we got into the first couple of chapters of the lessons, the Pirate showed no interest in doing any of the things Gary was asking us to do.

She seemed disinterested and was checking her Facebook all morning. I was trying not to get annoyed, but it was hard.

I was there to show that I was committed to this, and she was not into it.

At the break, I asked her if she was ok, and she talked about the time her husband and her were doing the same thing, and that the conference was triggering all those memories in her.

I asked if she wanted to leave, and she said no, she wanted to see if there was anything new added to the program in the last fifteen years ago.

She really wanted to hear about the chapter on sex and marriage.

So, after lunch, we got back into it, and the exercise came up that asked you to each write down what you were doing to make the relationship not work. Time to look at yourself and see what you could do better.

She didn't even write anything down. She threw the paper and the pen on the pew and got back on her Facebook.

I gave up. I put everything down and told her "let's go."

We got back to the car and drove towards St Augustine. I was very quiet for a while, and she knew I was upset. She asked me what was wrong, and I said the first thing that came to my mind,

"You know you just did to me what your husband did to you 15 years ago, don't you?"

She was upset by me not understanding that she had bad feelings brought on by the conference, and I eventually calmed down and tried to salvage the weekend. We spent the next two days in St. Augustine, but it was tense. When we got back to her home, we talked things out, and agreed that we should go to counseling to work these issues out.

We went to therapy every week for the next two months, but things were never the same. Every time I went to therapy, the Therapist would ask me if I was sure I wanted to be with a woman like the Pirate.

He explained how men and women were all on a spectrum. For a woman, most of them were on one side of the spectrum, where they need intimacy and emotional connection to have sex with a man.

He explained how the Pirate was on the opposite end of the spectrum. She saw sex as just a fun way to pass the time. She could sleep with many men, and never need a connection, or even a reason.

On the spectrum of men, most of them were on the end where it was just biology. They could sleep with as many women as they wanted with no emotional connection.

I, on the other hand, was on the opposite side of the spectrum, where I needed the emotions.

So, the Pirate and I were completely opposite, and he saw me getting extremely hurt by her. Which I eventually was.

It took many more arguments about me not trusting her, and she started giving me more and more reasons to not trust. By the beginning of April, I couldn't do it anymore. The final straw was a night we decided to spend apart, and she not only lied about where she was, and who she was with, but gave me a great opportunity to break up with her, which I did.

It was painful, but I have learned through all of this to walk away from anything that upsets my mental health.

I'm even worse at it now. I will erase people without hesitation. I just don't have the time or energy to make it work anymore. There's no reason to stay in something that isn't as close to healthy and perfect as it can be.

A week after I broke it off with the Pirate, I met an amazing woman named Jane.

Jane changed my whole perspective, and my life. She is who I have alluded to when I have said no one really saw the real me until I was 40.

She was the reason I was taken to Florida. She was the lesson I had to learn to really seek out healing for all of this, and to get my life into a place where I was at peace and could have a normative relationship. If a relationship at all is God's plan for my life.

She was what I was searching for most of my life when it concerned relationships.

Jane was a lesson, and an experience that I will take with me to my dying day and be forever grateful to God that I knew her at all.

It was a fluke, God's hands involved, that we even met in the first place.

Jane changed everything. Or rather, my time with her changed everything.

211

Chapter 27

I know that this narrative has been mostly about my relationships, but I whole-heartedly believe that our relationships are the most life-changing things we have. They affect our day, they weigh on our minds most of the day, and they give us our identity.

As husbands and wives, fathers and mothers, sons and daughters, all titles we have as humans, are all defined by a relationship.

When I write my fiction books after this, they will all revolve around that notion, that relationships are what we surround ourselves with when we are laying on our deathbeds.

It's not our career, or our possessions, or even our experiences that are the most important things at the end. It's the people in our lives.

God said it Himself in Genesis when he created Eve to be a companion for Adam. He said, "It's not good for Man to be alone."

We are such social creatures. The bible talks a lot about how important relationships are, especially the one we have with Jesus.

A relationship is the key to Heaven.

Our whole lives are based on our relationships, and they affect us the most, for better or worse.

So, my life story is about my relationships. And the last one I was in, with Jane, affected me the most. And it was the shortest.

I will start from the beginning.

Two days after I broke up with the Pirate, I was sitting in my apartment, and not really enjoying being alone. I knew that I needed to get to a point where I was ok not being with someone, but I just needed someone to talk to.

I really think that is how all my relationships start. I just need someone there, to talk to, and to know that I exist.

I certainly didn't want to meet someone like the Pirate, so I didn't think Tinder was the way to meet someone extraordinary.

I thought, maybe I needed to use a site I pay for. I had seen the commercials for eHarmony, so I thought that would be a great place to start. It was expensive, but the algorithm it used paired you up with someone who was most compatible.

With science behind it, how could it go wrong?

So, as I was sitting alone in my apartment, needing someone to talk to, I took the time to fill out the questionnaire for eHarmony. It was intensive, and very detailed. It took me about an hour to fill out, and I specified my distance to meet people was 50 miles.

I remember putting that in the profile because I didn't think long distance relationships worked.

With a 50-mile radius, and all the questions about myself and my preferences answered, I gave it to the dating site to find me Mrs. Right.

Three days later, I was matched with a woman named Jane. I sent her a little wave on April 15th. I remember that, because it was my brother's birthday, and we had plans for dinner that night.

Jane didn't respond until the next day, and we started slowly talking. The first night, it was maybe a dozen texts on the dating site. I asked her how to properly say her full name. She asked me what I did for a living. I told her, and she told me she was a therapist. Mostly dealing with relationships. She did a lot of couple's counseling.

Well now, I thought. Here was someone I could talk to. I was talking to four or five women on there at this point, so I didn't think much about her, other than I thought she was beautiful in her profile, and I was surprised how much we matched up on our answers to all the questions. We ranked almost 100% compatible on many factors.

So, after saying goodnight that night, I sent a little hello here and there over the next couple of weeks. I really went slowly. I was still talking to a couple of women, so she didn't stand out too much. It was incredibly casual, and very healthy.

At the same time, I was getting used to being alone, and started enjoying doing my own thing without having to worry about someone else's feelings, ideas, or issues. I was still going to the gym all the time, and work was going well.

I had nights where I went out with my buddies, and spent more time with my brother, who had moved to West Palm the month before.

I had a life that didn't revolve around a relationship, and I spent a lot of time alone in my apartment, catching up on shows I wanted to watch, and cooking meals just for myself.

If I had people to talk to on text, I wasn't lonely. It was an incredibly healthy time for me, and I think Jane saw that.

As the weeks went by, Jane and I started talking more and more. I found out that she lived in Ft. Myers, which was two and a half hours away. I wondered how we were even matched, as I knew that my radius was only 50 miles.

I asked her, and she had done the same. There was no way that we should have ever met, but here we were, talking, more than 200 miles apart.

I saw God's hand in that.

After two weeks of talking through the eHarmony site, I gave her my phone number. She still waited another week before using my number. We started texting more and more. We told each other our schedules, and we knew when each other would be available to chat.

The other women I was talking to dropped off, sometimes unexpectedly, and the time I spent talking to Jane began to increase.

Eventually we talked on the phone, and everything changed after that. There started to be days that we would talk almost all day, first on text, then phone calls when we were in bed at night that would last for hours.

The first time we talked for 8 hours straight, I knew that she was something special.

We connected on almost everything. Within a month of talking, we wanted to meet, and by then we had both completely fallen for each other's minds.

We had so many shared experiences and valued all the same things. And her being a therapist, she helped me establish healthy boundaries and topics to talk about.

Even then, we could have a conversation that lasted for hours, that felt like minutes, and which we both knew all the underlying issues neither of us were openly saying.

I came to know her on every level, before we even met, and she knew me. Our connection was deeper than any other I have ever had.

She reminded me of Ruth, from when I was 18. She was pure, and an amazing Christian woman. I trusted her instinctively.

215

She was the polar opposite of the pirate. It was amazingly easy to get to know her because it was like talking to myself. I learned and accepted that she came from a difficult background, a lot like mine, but she had risen above it and made something of herself, like I yearned to do as well.

She had persevered through a tough marriage and had two great kids. She came from nothing, had put herself through school, and worked harder than any other woman I knew. She had a bachelors and a masters and was certified by the state. Then, she went on to open her own practice, and eventually opened a second location.

Her business was growing, her kids were needing her less and less, and she was ready to be in a real relationship. I opened to her completely, sharing every difficult thing in my life, and was completely honest with her for the first time in my life.

I wasn't being untruthful with her as a defense mechanism this time. I told her every bad thing I had ever done and told her everything that is in this book.

She would be the one to eventually encourage me to write all of this and see if it was something people would want to read.

We began to send each other sweet, enduring texts that we would both wake up to. She started to be on my mind all the time, and I was on hers as well.

After a month of talking every day and getting to know each other as much as we could, we decided to finally meet.

As I didn't have a car at the time, she decided to come to West Palm. She drove two and a half hours to meet a man she had never met before. I can't imagine her nervousness, but she did it.

I made plans to meet her at a resort in West Palm Beach called the Eau Spa. It was a beautiful place. I got there early and had a drink at the whiskey bar.

I wore a shirt that fit me snuggly, because I was proud of my new body, and I wanted her to see me as I was now. She was aware of my weight loss and built me up and complimented me on it all the time. She knew about Prissy, and the Pirate.

She disliked both women.

When she walked into the Spa, I lost my breath. She was even more beautiful than her pictures. She literally lit up the room. We took a couple of pictures together because I wanted to record our first meeting.

This was a woman I knew I could spend the rest of my life with, and I had learned that over the last month of talking.

We had decided ahead of time that we weren't going to have sex this first weekend together. We didn't want to cloud our meeting. We knew we were extremely attracted to each other, but we didn't want the pressure.

I was fine with that and knew that we needed to establish our identity in each other first. But don't be alarmed, she was incredibly sexy, and I was smitten with her.

When we met, I had a small gift bag full of things I thought she would like. I always try to have a gift. I was brought up that way.

She walked in holding a small gift bag as well. It was full of my favorite Easter candy, Cadbury caramel eggs.

It was an obscure fact I had told her a month earlier and she ordered the candy online and brought me a whole bag of them.

It was incredibly touching, and I didn't know she had planned that for me.

We spent the weekend together. We slept in the same bed at night, without having sex. It was all so easy, and comfortable.

We clicked on every level, and there wasn't anything about her I didn't like.

On Sunday afternoon, while napping together, we did get a little physical. I wanted to see what she looked like naked, and got to do that, after a lot of playing and teasing. I was very dominating, and I think she liked that. I assured she was comfortable with it all, though. She was adorably shy about her body, but she was perfect.

She saw me naked as well and told me that she was pleasantly surprised. I knew that going forward, after we got that part out of the way, it would be a lot easier to establish the physical part of our relationship.

We ended up putting a lot of pressure on sex when we were finally intimate a few weeks later, but it got better the longer we were together. We were both such intellectual people, and are ruled by our minds, that we overthink everything.

It's to be expected, but we were both doing it, and somehow, we were building each other up, and being strong for each other when the other needed it. It just all worked perfectly in the beginning.

There was a time, early on, when she started pulling away because she found it was something she did with every relationship she has been in.

I felt so strong for her during those weeks.

I was dependable, understanding, and stood by her. I didn't get freaked out and take it personally like I would have done in the past. She made me feel whole, and like a real man. Being able to be honest with her and share myself with her freed me to be strong for her when she needed me to be.

I later messed it all up, but at that moment, I was the perfect man for her.

We eventually shared our mutual love for each other. I told her on the phone how I felt about her, two and a half hours apart, thinking it was the worse way to tell someone you were falling in love with them, but she answered me right back.

She said,

"J.L., I am in love with you too. I know I love you."

She used my name and was so sincere I almost cried. I was so damn happy. A lot of people would say that we rushed that part. It had only been six weeks since we met, but I will tell you now, I would have said it to her the second week.

I fell for her hard, from the beginning. And it wasn't her body, or her sexiness, which a lot of men put such big importance

. It was her mind, our shared connection, and experiences, and who she was. I thought for the first time in my life that I had met the perfect woman for me.

I hadn't felt anything like that since I was 18, and that paled to this. This was so adult and grown up and healthy.

We talked about absolutely everything, and when we would get together on the weekends, it was even better. We had both a mental and a physical connection.

But it wasn't all roses and cupcakes. We were both products of our pasts, and both of us freaked out a bit on each other. She was much healthier about it than I was.

One area we had negative discussions about was her children. I had left my long-term family unit the year before and missed it tremendously.

When I was over her house, I got too comfortable and her older daughter had a wrong impression of me. Jane told me that she and her daughter were unhealthily co-dependent on each other, and she was working on that, but I was not a good thing to come into that situation and upset it.

219

I really had the best of intentions, but that was one area I rushed. I never met her 11-year-old daughter. We were waiting to make sure that we were together forever before I would meet her youngest daughter, and I just would get frustrated because when she had her youngest, it meant that I couldn't see her.

I pushed a little too hard a couple of times in that regard, and it really soured Jane on me. We recovered the times we spoke about it, but it was a huge red flag for her that I was concerned in that area.

I really did push too hard in the family department. I shouldn't have, and I know that now. That was a part of Jane's life she wasn't ready to share, and I made a lot of mistakes trying to insinuate myself in her whole life.

I learned a major lesson in that area. Those things are sacred, and I know now that it wasn't my business in that regard.

It wouldn't be for more than a year since we met, that's what we agreed on, but we didn't make it that far.

Everything was going so well with us though. We were really getting close. Closer than I had gotten with any other woman in my life. She really was perfect in so many ways.

She wasn't a perfect person; she was just perfect for me. I tried to be that for her, I really did. It was all going so well, and we were so deep into each other, and then my birthday happened.

The events that transpired from the beginning of June to the beginning of August would forever change everything about me, and who I am.

This book is dedicated to those 8 weeks. Everything that has transpired in this book, the whole forty years, led up to those 8 weeks.

I will be forever altered by those 8 weeks.

I would hit the bottom of a hole deeper than anything I ever knew before, and it would be because of everything that has ever happened to me, coming back all at once.

And then God would pull me out like he has so many times before.

I sit here now, a month removed from those 8 weeks, more than a thousand miles away from where they happened, finally, finally at peace.

And between me and God, nobody got me there. There isn't a relationship in the world strong enough to fix what has transpired in this book so far.

The peace I have now is from God, and nothing from here on out will ever take this away from me again.

I will fight for this harder than anything else in my life.

I am alone in life right now, and I am completely fine. I am happier, have more joy, and sleep well at night without needing another person in my life.

Completeness has not come from another person, finally. I don't look for a relationship, for the first time in my life, to find peace and purpose. God has shown me to look within, to forgive myself completely, and to love the only person who I can truly depend on. Me. Nothing will ever steal my joy again.

The rest of this book will detail those 8 weeks between June and August, 2019.

And they were like nothing that came before. Not even close.

Chapter 28

My fortieth birthday came in the first week of June, as it's known to do. This year, my birthday would fall on a Monday, so the weekend before, Jane and I met in Miami to celebrate.

We threw back and forth ideas for a lot of our friends to join us, but in the end, I decided that I just wanted to spend some time alone with her.

She had a previous engagement to attend to that weekend. A training for her continuing education. It took place on Friday afternoon, and Saturday morning in Miami.

She had already set up a hotel room, so I just drove there on Friday afternoon, and met her in the room after her class. We took a shower together, something we tried to do as much as possible, and made love deep into the afternoon.

That night, we ordered in food, and spent many nice, quiet hours together. We talked deep into the night and held each other until we fell asleep. The month before, we had professed our love for each other, and had been through some ups and downs leading up to this weekend together.

I had made a playlist of music on my streaming music app, and I played it all that afternoon. We completely lost ourselves in each other, and for the first time in a very long time, with any woman, I was able to orgasm inside of her. That wall took a lot to break down.

It never fully came down, and still hasn't, but it showed me that I completely trusted this woman. I trusted her with my heart, and my emotional and mental wellbeing.

I thought she could handle it, but it was too much to ask of anyone. Even someone who was perfect for me and handled people in crisis every day in her job.

The weekend flew by in a blink, and we got to know each other deeper than we had before. We spoke honestly with each other about things we were afraid to bring up before then.

I learned things about her that I didn't necessarily like, but I was in love with her, and nothing would change that.

Small tendrils of mistrust started creeping into my mind from the brutally honest conversations we had that weekend, sitting in that nicely appointed hotel room in Miami.

Those small tendrils would become humongous snakes of deep-seated mental instability within a month.

When the weekend was finished, and I drove back to my apartment in West Palm Beach, doubts started creeping into the nicely carved out image I had of Jane.

It wasn't anything big or horrible that started the slow decline. It was the fact that she didn't live up to my over-inflated expectations.

Which was completely unfair to her.

I could see that this was something that I had done with many women. They don't meet my completely unfair opinions, and I start to pull away from them.

223

I didn't think too much about it, still being more in love with her than any other woman I knew in my life. I felt emotions for her that scared me, and frankly, I had not felt with anyone else.

I had been married three times, and none of the emotions I felt for those three women stood up to the level of love I felt for Jane. Mix those feelings with what happened in my life in the next two months, and not even a saint would have stayed with me.

The day of my actual birthday dawned bright. I had gotten up early for work and went in at my normal time of 5am. I took a picture in the mirror in my bathroom before I left for the day. I posted it on social media and was proud of the fact that I was in better shape at 40 than I had been since high school.

In the evening, after going to the gym and my normal routine, I was sitting, alone, watching television.

Jane had texted me throughout the day and knew that I was emotional because I was alone.

There was a knock on my door. I answered it and saw a pizza deliveryman standing there. He asked me if it was my birthday, and I said yes, and he sang me the birthday song, and then handed me a hot, large pizza.

I set it on the kitchen counter and opened it. It had my favorite toppings on it, but on top of that there was a heart made out of pepperoni.

I called Jane right away and found out that she had set the whole thing up with the pizza joint. I thanked her repeatedly and she listened as I ate several slices.

My day was instantly made better, and I fell asleep that night knowing that I was lonely but was extremely lucky. I had an amazing woman who loved me.

That night was the last time I felt any positive emotions for the next two months.

On the 11th of the month, I got laid off of my job. No warning, no way to prepare. Just let go. This event precipitated a crazy dive into a hole that was deeper than any I had ever been in.

Two days later, my roommate at my apartment informed me that he would be moving in with his boyfriend on July 1st, and I had to be out of the apartment by then.

I had no recourse, and no options. Within a week, I lost my job and my home.

Three weeks later, I would be homeless, and with very few options, would be sleeping in my car on the weekends, in a Walmart parking lot, in the middle of a Florida summer.

On June 20th, right before her 41st birthday, Jane and I had a huge argument when I pushed to meet her kids. I thought that if I met her children, then the times that she was with them wouldn't exclude me anymore.

I just wanted more time with her, and I justified it by arguing with her. She disagreed, and I think she was seeing the spiral I was in because of where my life was going.

I left the weekend of her birthday a day earlier than I had planned and drove back to West Palm Beach.

On the drive back, Jane called me and told me that she had been feeling off the whole weekend because of the argument we had.

She knew that I had been feeling off because she was off. She told me that she needed some time to think, and that she would contact me when she had given it enough time to figure out how she felt.

That was Sunday morning. The next day, starting on June 24th, I came to realize that I had completely ruined my life, again.

I started to spiral, and that week is labeled in my calendar as "The WEEK".

I woke up after only getting less than 2 hours of sleep the previous two nights, on Tuesday morning, and I broke up with Jane over text message.

Later the next afternoon, I was on Reddit, reading stories about people going through depression.

Someone posted a question on u/AskReddit that basically said, "What's scaring you right now?" I posted the following, word for word:

"Right now, everything is happening all at once.

1. *I have to be out of my apartment by July 1st. My roommate, who has the lease decided last month to move in with his boyfriend and gave me 4 weeks to move out of the apartment I've been in for a year.*

2. *June 11th, I got laid off of my job. I have been in military aviation in one way or another for 22 years, since joining the Air Force at 18. I have received no replies from the 50+ jobs I've applied to.*

3. *I broke up with the woman who I thought was perfect and who I totally love yesterday because she ghosted me after a conversation we had on her birthday on Friday about moving on to the next level. I broke up with her because I felt like she was going to break up with me and after a childhood of horrible trauma and being an orphan, I run before people can hurt me. I have worked on this in counseling, but I know I need more therapy.*

4. *I only have about 700 dollars to make it until I get another job and since the plan was to move to the city my gf lives, I am not doing that now. So, in one week I will be homeless without a job.*

5. *I have been praying to God for a month to lead me in the right direction, but I haven't felt him guiding me, nor has anything happened to show me the way. I feel completely alone. I'm so lonely this week. I have been in my apartment since Sunday, applying to jobs but not hearing anything back at all. I have a few friends, but it's been my girlfriend who I have been closest to this year and now I've ruined that. I have struggled all my life, fought my way through trial after trial, always in poverty, always having to do everything myself with no support. I have no family except a brother, who is awesome, but is also busy far away getting started in a new level of his career. He is beyond blessed in his life, and he doesn't believe in God.*

I guess what I'm saying is, please pray for me. I'm praying for a miracle right now. I'm putting it all in God's hands, which I believe is how I've gotten through life so far, even though it's always been a struggle. I'm so tired of fighting. I'm just so tired. There is much more to the story, like my two divorces, my children I can't support right now, and how I got my car repossessed, and since moving to Florida, I have been making half what I made in Maryland, so I have fallen further and further behind. My credit score has tanked, and I don't even know if I could get my security clearance back if I move back to Maryland for government contractor work, which is what I've done for the last 12 years.

Again, I'm just so tired.... I feel like giving it all up. I don't know how much strength I have left. It's all so damn heavy. And I'm going to finish it off this week, one way or another."

Dated June 26, 2019.

Chapter 29

And so, you, constant reader, are up to date on what transpired next. I was going to kill myself, I was at peace, and as I prepared to finish the job, I called my best friend, Mary Elizabeth, who told me to call Jasper.

So, after I calmed down, I called Jasper. He was in town, and said that he had some stuff to do, but that he wanted us to get together that evening and go see a movie. I had not been outside of my apartment for a week except to walk around my neighborhood. I felt like I hadn't had a shower the whole time. I felt like I needed to clean myself up.

I walked into the bathroom and I looked a mess. I hadn't shaved or slept much. I hadn't eaten all week, and I looked gaunt. I looked like a ghost of myself. My eyes were bloodshot, my skin pale.

I took off my loose clothes and climbed into the hot shower. I stayed in there until well after the water turned cold. I felt the hot water wash over my skin, and I started to feel clean.

But it was the feeling of cleanliness on the inside. I knew that my road ahead was going to be tough, but I didn't have anyone to blame anymore. I knew talking to Jasper that evening would be hard, but it, too, would be cleansing.

My road, over the last 14 months, had been completely up and down, crazy at times, but looking back from that day, and especially where I am sitting right now, there was a reason for all of it.

It was the biggest transformational time in my life since I went to Boys Ranch.

I learned things about myself in those months in Florida that would once again shape me into a different person. The second stage of my life was now over. The first had ended with my transformation in the Spirit, in that jail cell in Utah. This second stage had ended in the same hole I had been in then.

I was much closer to ending it this time than I was the first time, but I could plainly see the road I had traveled.

In the book of James in the bible, it tells us to ask God for wisdom, and He gives it in spades. But we cannot doubt when we ask for wisdom, because that would make us like a wave tossed on the ocean.

I had certainly been awash on a sea of pain and wrong decisions. No one was to blame for where I was in my life, but as I stood once again in front of that mirror after my cleansing shower, dried off and feeling much better about myself, I again asked God for wisdom.

And He did a wonderful thing.

He reminded me that He had given me a gift. My main gift. A gift of words. I heard His still small voice in my mind telling me,

"Ok, now it's time to tell this story."

That evening, sitting in my brother's truck, I laid out the whole week to him, and what I had planned. He hit me in the back of my head so hard it hurt his oversized hand. I shuddered and cried again, and he was shaken because he had never seen me cry before. He stopped on the way to the movies, and in his own way, did what he thought was best for me. He bought us both ice cream.

We ate it as we walked into the movies, and again, I felt the love that God had shown me that morning had always been there.

Jasper put his big meaty arms around me and pulled me close, hugging me in the way only your big brother can hug you, and I loved him even more for that gesture.

229

For the next four weeks, he would help me tremendously, and when I finally made the changes in my life that I needed to make, for me, he was there to wish me the best, and see me off.

He told me that he knew that good things would happen for me. I just had to learn what I learned there in Florida, before I could go on to the next chapter, and whatever that would hold.

I couldn't believe how much God was going to bless me. And how fast he would make it all work out.

I truly came through the valley of the shadow of death, and it was love that had brought me through.

Chapter 30

Before I met up with Jasper that evening, I texted Jane. I asked her if she would give me some of her time, to come to where she lived, meet somewhere quiet, and let me tell her some truths. She agreed, and we planned to meet at a tiki bar near a river.

I got to the place the next day early. I had to gather my thoughts. I didn't know what the future held, but I knew that I need to tell Jane the whole story of the past. I especially had to tell her about the last week of my life.

I was sitting at a table near the water, and the beautiful boats tied up at the long dock. There was a small breeze, but it was hot. I was wearing a nice shirt and shorts, and I saw her walking towards me wearing a thin summer dress.

She had put on makeup and looked amazing. I still felt my chest catch looking at her.

I knew that I felt love for her. I never doubted that the emotions I had for her were some that I had walled myself away from feeling for so many years, and for so many relationships.

She sat at the table across from me and we both ordered a beer and a water. I always loved how she ordered anything at a restaurant. She was so exact, and knew exactly what she wanted, and how she wanted it. Some would get annoyed at her multi-leveled order for something as simple as iced tea, but I loved it about her.

I laughed every time we had been on the phone while she went through a drive-thru to order anything. I had memorized her order from different places.

As our beers arrived, I took a deep breath, looked her square in the eyes, and told her absolutely everything that is in this story.

She had not known about Sara until that day.

She did not know about my contemplated suicide at the age of 26, or the one only the day before.

She didn't know about the years between Victoria and Prissy where I went crazy with how many women I slept with.

I laid it all out over the next three hours.

The beers got warm while we talked, never touching our drinks. The words poured out of me, and as they did, the stirrings of a desire to write this all down quickened in my heart.

She listened as only a therapist can listen, asking details and clarifications as I rambled on and on. She would reach across the table and take my hand during the hard parts, like my time at the boy's home in California, and the nightly rapes I had endured at the hands of the older boys.

I had kept these things from her because I had learned that they can scare away a new relationship. But she listened and accepted, and I could see the love in her eyes.

It was getting dark by the time I finished the tale. We walked out to the cars in the deserted parking lot, and she asked me for a kiss and to hold her for a little bit.

I did just that.

I pulled her in close, smelling her smell, and feeling her heartbeat against my stomach.

I knew she loved me. I knew I loved her.

I didn't know where we went from there, but I knew I wanted to be with her. My life was in an absolute shit heap at the moment, but I wanted to be with her in whatever way she would have me.

We parted ways, promising to talk soon.

I called her the next day with a new plan.

My brother had been working in Ft. Myers, where she lived, and he invited me to stay with him during the weekdays while he was in a hotel and working. On the weekends he would go to his house in West Palm Beach, and I would have to find somewhere to stay. He assumed that I would stay with Jane, and I did, but only a couple of times when both of her children were gone.

As it was my brother's idea to move, he helped me by giving me money to move with, and to have a little left over to live on for a while.

So, I went back to West Palm Beach and packed up my apartment. I had until July 4th to move out, and it was on that day that I said goodbye to West Palm Beach and the little over a year I had been there. There was no send off, no goodbye dinner with friends. I simply drove away.

When I got to Ft. Myers it started going downhill fast.

I was now in Jane's hometown, and the reality of how close I was to her hit her hard. She was not ready for the intensity and angst I would display over the next month.

The only work I could find quickly was delivering pizzas in North Ft. Myers. I did this almost every day. It was ok money, but never enough to get on my own.

I would stay the week in the hotel with my brother, and when he left on the weekends, if I didn't have enough money saved up for the weekend room rates, I slept in my car in a Walmart parking lot.

I couldn't roll the windows down because of the constant swarms of bugs, so I baked in the car. I would turn the ignition on several times during the night to cool the inside of the car off a little, but it was never enough.

I continued to lose weight, and my depression got worse. And I took it all out on Jane.

She tried to maintain a healthy relationship with me, but I pushed and pushed her beyond her breaking point.

During this month, she even showed more of her amazing character by offering me a job. I could use my experience and knowledge to help her business, and she, in turn would not only pay me, but also help me get my certification to be a life coach.

I could rent a space from her, and she would start referring clients to me that she felt would benefit from my particular brand of lifting other's up and increasing their moral.

I researched it heavily that month, but by the end of July, she had had enough of my nightly resentment texts that I would send because she had a home and a family and friends, and I was so alone still so much of the time.

My mental health did not improve that month, but my resolve to do something about it did.

I just needed a catalyst.

On August 3rd, almost a month since moving to Ft. Myers for what I thought was my new beginning, and that catalyst came in the form of an email while I was delivering pizzas.

One of the things that I really wanted to start doing during my time in Ft. Myers was to write this story. I didn't know how it would end, only that I needed to start it.

I started writing it in the worse place of my life, on July 5th.

I was just going to put it on paper. It was a need and a drive I felt deep within myself.

I would go every day before delivering pizzas to the local coffee shop to sit and write a couple of chapters, just getting it all out.

I sent it to be read by a couple of close friends, including Graham and Jane and Mary. Everyone supported me in writing this, and I was excited to see where it would go. What I didn't expect, is that while I was writing it, all the old feelings I had from all those experiences would come back to haunt me, and would reflect on how I interacted with Jane, and how I treated her.

I know that I did everything wrong that I could in that month. I thought I was gaining mental health, but the truth was, I was living back in the past, and it was affecting my future. Putting all of these experiences down on paper made me relive all of those emotions I thought I had gotten through in therapy. But I was wrong. I needed a last catalyst, a final change, to be able to process all of this. I'm sure you, as you read these pages, have had emotions. Imagine living though it all.

I didn't know how bad it was for Jane, who tried with everything she could to love me through it, but in the end, she had to do what was the best for her, and for her own mental and emotional health.

I finally pushed too far. And she pushed right back.

The previous week before August 3rd, Jane and I had decided to have a date night that we hoped would turn into a weekly event.

I picked her up from work and had bought salami's and cheeses to make a picnic on her favorite beach.

I bought a bottle of wine and we made it to the beach just in time to see the beautiful sunset behind the Gulf of Mexico. It started out as an amazing night, and of course, I had to mess it all up with my insecurity and mistrust.

Driving back, I once again mentioned meeting her daughter, and that I wanted to meet her so that I could be with Jane more often.

It wasn't a survival ploy, just so I would have somewhere to stay, it was a yearning for the family that I had been without for the last year.

She got her defenses up as she had done the weekend of her birthday. I ended up dropping her off at her house, and she asked for time to think about how she felt about things. I didn't hear from her for a week. When I did, it was in the form of the following email:

Hey there,

I wanted to send an email because it's easier to write. So, I have been thinking about the past three and a half months. I do agree with you that in the beginning and throughout there were times when we got along great. I agree that I had feelings stir up at certain points. I also saw in the texts that I consistently tried to slow things down and for good reasoning. Going through a divorce after being in a family unit is a traumatic event, as you know. I'm not even sure that I am ready to be in a serious relationship and after reading the last three chapters of your book, it is very clear that you are not ready for sure. There is a reason why we have been on a roller coaster and the reasons really don't matter, what is evident is that we are not able to be in a relationship. I don't have what it takes to be in this relationship, and it is very clear to me that you don't either. I'm too old, been through too much and have way too much going on to try to navigate this. It is not healthy for me. I won't speak for you. You have to figure that out.

I would still like to be friends if that's possible. I think that I could be just a friend, but I don't know if you can. I would still like for us to work together as well, but again, I don't know if you can do that without being in a romantic relationship. We would have to talk about all of this to see if it were a possibility. I sign on the new office today and have to be out of the Bonita office this weekend.

I hope you are doing well. I know that you are a good person J.L. and have great potential professionally and as a partner in a relationship (when you are healed and in a better place emotionally). It's clear from what you have said that you're still healing from your divorce and your childhood. Let me know if you would like to meet up and talk.

Jane

I wasn't surprised or upset to receive that email. I called her, and as I was delivering a pizza a few blocks from her house, asked if I could come over and get my dog tags, which I had given to her when we first met.

She answered the door and handed me my tags. I tried my best to find the words to apologize, but they didn't come out right. For being a person trained in using words to tell exactly what I wanted to tell, I couldn't arrange them in any coherent way that day. We texted back and forth a couple of times in the weeks after that, but it got nowhere. She had moved on, and that was the healthiest thing for her to do. It would take me much longer to move on, but her breaking up with me was exactly what I needed to make the next moves in my life. To get myself together and make some decisions.

I was a free man again. Free to make my own choices and not be weighted down with the responsibility of a relationship and all the pressure I put on them every time.

The day after she broke up with me, I woke up with a new purpose. That next Monday, I applied for five Tech Writing jobs back in Maryland and prayed to God to make something happen if that was His will.

Within the week, I had five interviews, and I was hired on the spot from the phone interview I had on Thursday of that next week.

On Friday of that week, two weeks to the day that Jane had broken up with me, I was on the road back to Maryland.

I had enough money to make it there and start over. I had called my best friend Danny back in Southern Maryland, and he agreed to let me stay with him.

As I drove away from Florida, the rain that had fallen every day for the last two months dried up, a rainbow showed itself right in front of my car, and I smiled once again to myself. I could feel the invisible cord of memory connecting me to the person I was when I first drove down to Florida, on the same stretch of road.

It was 15 months to the day since I left Maryland for something, I felt, God was leading me to. And I knew beyond any disbelief that He gave me the lessons I had to learn.

The pirate had been a huge lesson. And Jane had been the blessing that God led me down south for.

Jane had shown me one single thing. That there were wonderful, beautiful people in this life that could and would love me, and that I could finally let down the walls to love in return.

I drove back to Maryland lighthearted and happy. I didn't know what the future held, but the entire test and trial I had to go through to get back on that road 15 months later had been well worth it.

I found my peace as the tires of my car crunched on the blacktop. I got to the top of the hill separating Florida and Georgia, and I felt that invisible line of memory snap.

I turned my head forward, felt two tears drop from my eyes, and pressed the gas pedal.

I drove towards my new future, alone.

And I didn't looked back.

Chapter 31

I want to take a moment here and talk about what this book is about, why I wrote it, and what I hope to do with it. I want to talk about my diagnosis, and what it means, not only in my life, but in the choices I have made, and continue to make.

I recently watched a TedTalk, from the now-Surgeon General in the state of California, Nadine Burke Harris, and I had such a "Eureka" moment.

Everything this esteemed doctor spoke about, specifically how Adverse Childhood Experiences affect adult life, made me realize that this story needed to be told.

I did not do the best job of describing the abuse and neglect I went through as a child. I don't know that I can ever speak to the real details. The fear, the stress, the everyday feelings of fight or flight. All my young life was in some way or another the reason why I have made the decisions, and am affected by physical problems I now have, for my whole life.

I know now that I need to not only tell this story but to do everything I can to inform the public about this growing, and horribly dangerous trend we now have in the mental health fields.

Complex Post Traumatic Stress Disorder is a fairly new diagnosis for a very old issue. There are a few treatment options for those diagnosed with this disorder, but many who suffer from this diagnosis, even when it is properly diagnosed, cannot afford, or even find caregivers that are trained to properly care for these individuals.

When I first discovered my diagnosis, I started doing a lot of research, as I'm keen on doing. This book started out as a means to tell my story, and as a therapy tool for myself. I didn't have a true idea of what it would become, or where it would go.

Since finishing it, it has become something entirely different. I am going to move forward with publishing this book for one sole purpose.

To shine a spotlight on an uncomfortable realization.

That there are thousands and tens of thousands of children whose very lives and futures are irreparably disrupted because of abuse perpetrated on them by those they trusted.

This abuse WILL affect the outcome of every area of their adult life because their normal development was disrupted in a dramatic way.

I like the way that Dr. Harris described how the brain of an affected child works.

Pretend you're walking through a forest and there is a bear. Your brain jumps into action. Signals go to your glands that release hormones that inflate your muscular response. Your pupils dilate, your lungs expand for more oxygen. You are physically ready to choose to fight that bear or run from that bear. Which is a beautiful thing. One of the miracles of our bodies.

But what if that bear comes home every night?

What if your body, and your brain goes to that overdrive response every single day?

Can you imagine how prolonged use of that "miracle" of our physical bodies can have traumatic effects later in life?

And that is just the physical response. Can you imagine the emotional response of all of that fear? The mistrust; frankly, the panic and horror.

Our caregivers are supposed to be the main people we can rely on to take care of us when we can't do it ourselves. How do you survive when that caregiver abuses you in ways that take decades to overcome?

I urge everyone to look up Dr. Harris's TedTalk on the matter of Adverse Childhood Experiences. It's quite eye-opening. And now, she is in a position to do a lot of really good change in the state that all of my abuses happened.

At the end of this book I'm going to list resources where anyone can go to find out their own system of recovery, as well as personal tests that you can take to get an initial idea of where you stand in your own mental health, and where you should go to seek help for the way it is affecting your everyday life.

If you have found yourself un-controllably doing some of the things listed below in your job, your relationships, your interactions with others, please seek whatever help you can. We have to get the spotlight on how these issues are affecting us as a human race.

Early prevention and education have shown to lower the long-term effects of childhood abusive disorders. But it's an extremely sensitive subject, as the majority of the abuse happening to children are done by those closest to them, and the adults do not either realize they have become perpetrators of child abuse, or they refuse to seek help for their own issues before passing the same affectivities to the children around them.

Below, I have included an excerpt from the website www.beautyafterbruises.org. When I read the following for the first time, I nearly crumbled. I realized that I have done, and continue to do, the following reactive events in every aspect of my adult life.

Every single one.

As I started this book, I innocently stated that I feel completely alien from all those around me. And I thought I was alone in feeling that way. But here, finally, was the reason that I am the way I am.

And the first step in my recovery was accepting that it wasn't my fault that I have reacted this way. But it was my fault that I never sought out proper treatment for this, as it was even affecting my children.

My oldest son, Graham, has recently communicated to me his own issues with depression and emotional de-regulation. I have done everything I can for him to seek help on his own. It's now up to him, as a twenty-one-year-old adult, to use those resources to try and fix the issues he has stemming from his own childhood.

A childhood I had a huge hand in shaping, and ultimately helping to enact similar abuses on him, and my other children, unbeknownst to me.

So, as I studied and wrote this book, I realized my recovery wasn't just for myself or my future relationships, but also for my children. And their children.

Even today, I have noticed my behavior in my new relationships. I start pushing away and being hyper vigilant with them, which they do not deserve at all.

And I am only hurting them, and myself.

I hate the feelings I have when I do not allow the therapeutic tools I have learned to use every day to take the place of the triggers of my diagnosis.

I only pray someone can stick it out with me, through the peaks and valleys to come, and see me for something other than how I see myself.

I believe, deep in my heart, that I am worth it. I hope one day someone else will as well. And I hope that I can be strong enough to help them through their own troubles.

In the meantime, I am going to weekly therapy and learning to keep loving myself. I am just going to stop trying to date. I haven't even met anyone in real life. Just talking on the phone, and I'm already pushing. The women don't tell me that, but I can see it in myself, and feel it.

It's going to take one hell of a woman to try to understand and appreciate who I am and what I offer and see past the triggers I still have.

Or maybe not see past them, but try to not take them personally, and to understand this most of all: I crave unconditional love more than anything.

I am also lucky in my faith. God has had a huge hand in shaping who I am today, and while not yet whole, better than I should be. He has kept me alive. He has blessed me even when I daily rail and scream at Him for my unfair life. Through the relationships He has placed in my life, I am still here.

And He will have control of where this book, as well as the following books, go, and I pray it will be used for His purpose.

Following, is a very accurate description of what C-PTSD is, and how it blooms in adulthood:

"Complex PTSD comes in response to chronic traumatization over the course of months or, more often, years. This can include emotional, physical, and/or sexual abuses, domestic violence, living in a war zone, being held captive, human trafficking, and other organized rings of abuse, and more. While

there are exceptional circumstances where adults develop C-PTSD, it is most often seen in those whose trauma occurred in childhood. For those who are older, being at the complete control of another person (often unable to meet their most basic needs without them), coupled with no foreseeable end in sight, can break down the psyche, the survivor's sense of self, and affect them on this deeper level. For those who go through this as children, because the brain is still developing and they're just beginning to learn who they are as an individual, understand the world around them, and build their first relationships - severe trauma interrupts the entire course of their psychologic and neurologic-development

When an adult experiences a traumatic event, they have more tools to understand what is happening to them, their place as a victim of that trauma, and know they should seek support even if they don't want to. Children don't possess most of these skills, or even the ability to separate themselves from another's unconscionable actions. The psychological and developmental implications of that become complexly woven and spun into who that child believes themselves to be -- creating a messy web of core beliefs much harder to untangle than the flashbacks, nightmares and other posttraumatic symptoms that come later.

Another important thing to know is that the trauma to children resulting in C-PTSD (as well as dissociative disorders) is usually deeply interpersonal within that child's caregiving system. Separate from both the traumatic events and the perpetrator, there is often an added component of neglect, hot-and-cold affections from a primary caregiver, or outright invalidation of the trauma if a child does try to speak up. These disorganized attachments and mixed messages from those who are supposed to provide love, comfort, and safety - all in the periphery of extreme trauma - can create even more unique struggles that PTSD-sufferers alone don't always face.

245

(www.beautyafterbruises.org, 2019)

I urge you to visit this wonderful website and read the rest of the information. There is so much more than just that little bit.

And it explained everything I had ever done in my life. Every decision. Every hurt.

Reading these things has shown me that my treatment is far from over. Seeing what I still do every day makes me realize that my treatment is far from over. And it is all connected. Every action I make in my relationships today that stems from my abusive past makes me perpetrate the abuses again and again today.

Now, my partners unknowingly keep the abuse going, through no idea or thought of their own. It's because every action they take, based on my own actions, turns around and becomes more abuse to me.

It will take an extraordinarily strong woman to go through this with me. The biggest reason I do the things that I do in a relationship is because I have extremely low self-esteem. I fake confidence. And when I have gotten close to someone who responds to that confidence, I start to let the affectivities in, and push away the new relationship.

It is a self-fulfilling prophesy.

I have yet to meet a woman who can understand these things I do, and persevere through them to see the real me, especially when I can't see the real me myself. All I can do is work on my own treatment, and hope one day, that the experiences in my past, and the fear I have as a result of it, will stop affecting my future.

I am well on my way in recovery, but there is still so much work to do. As of the finishing of this book, I have been single for almost a year. I have learned to enjoy my time with myself, and I don't even know if I will ever have another relationship. I have hope for it, but it's God's Will. I am neither looking, nor pursuing anything in that regard.

But I am lucky. Extremely lucky. I'm still here. I am still surrounded by love. And I respond to that love. Like a man about to die in the desert, who comes across a pool of crystal clear, cold water. But I, as that dying man, must first spend a very long time convincing myself that I don't deserve the water, or that the water is really not there.

That, is the worse of the abuse. The fact that as an adult, I can realize that it happened, but I cannot control how it has affected those around me now. My abusers didn't only destroy my self-worth and sense of safety, but they destroyed the happiness I could have had with any number of women that have been in my life from years ago to now.

That fact makes me the saddest.

The resources at the end of this book, as well as the information found in those websites and hospitals will show that this is a larger issue in the world then what we want to accept.

There is less than a 1% chance of coverage for those dealing with these issues. The sad fact is, that much higher percentages of those affected by C-PTSD end up taking their own lives than any other demographic out there.

And it won't just affect those suffering from it. Studies have proven that those individuals with an ACE score (Adverse Childhood Experiences) have 8 to 10 times the likelihood of developing later-in-life medical issues like lung disease, heart disease, cancer, and suicide than any other demographic.

This is all a very real, reportable, and preventable issue. I heard one statistic that as age progresses of a +4 ACE score individual, their systemic medical issues stemming from those childhood experiences will become the next global medical pandemic.

We must make changes.

These numbers do not lie. And this book is one of many that highlight these realities. We MUST, as a combined global consciousness, not only put a stop to childhood abuses, but also reach out and help those dealing with these issues in their everyday lives as adults.

I urge anyone dealing with these afflictions to reach out, in any way they can, and start the process of learning to control their own lives.

I am on that journey now.

And, as I'll speak about at the closing of this book, I have a hope in my life now that pushes me to make these changes as soon, as hard, and as perfectly, as I can.

Chapter 32

So, here we are.

I am sitting once again in a coffee shop and looking around at the people. Everyone has problems. Everyone has relationships. Everyone is loved by God.

And so am I.

I am no different from the people around me. No more special. No less important. I belong with these people. I belong with all people.

I know now, that after everything in the last 40 years, I don't have to let it affect me or my future. That's between me and God, and He has done an amazing job of carrying me to this day, in this place, to finish this book.

So where is everyone now?

My brother Jasper continues to work and live in Florida. He is highly successful at his job, and makes an amazing living doing exactly what he loves doing. He has saved lives in his profession and moved up the ladder in astonishing speed.

He will continue to be my strongest supporter, and I would lay my life down in a heartbeat for him. We speak every day, and he has been my anchor in this life, no more so than the last 15 months. He always says that I am his "person," but the truth is, he is mine. He has been through everything with me, and I love him fiercely.

My sisters are all still spread out.

Zoie continues to work and live in Northern California, in the same neighborhood we lived in while my father was alive.

Harmony just made tenure at Job Corp, where she has taught for the last 15 years. She brings light to the world in ways that cannot be quantified. All of my siblings deserve to write their own stories, like I did here. My father dying in 1988 created lives in each of us that have been painful and extremely hard, but made us all so very strong.

Venus Layne, who I haven't mentioned much in this story, works in Ft. Lauderdale. She has been so very important in my life, without being directly in my life. I see her life and goals and beliefs spread out on social media every day.

She has had a much harder road to walk than the rest of us, but with strength and determination, she has always done everything she could to care for her children, and fight for what she believes in. She is truly a champion for the disadvantaged and downtrodden. She is an advocate for those treated less than, by the rest of the world. She rallies people to the causes of equality for everyone, no matter your choices in life, but she also fights for those choices, and that everyone has the unalienable right to any choice they see fit for their own lives.

I secretly admire her more than anyone else on this planet for her strength and conviction, and while I don't agree with everything she does, or says, I love her fiercely, all the same.

My kids are all doing very well. Graham dropped out of college after a year of working overtime to do everything that was expected of him. He will turn 21 next month and is working two jobs on his own now.

He just moved into an apartment in Lubbock, TX with his girlfriend, and besides being completely honest with me when we talk everyday about his depression and lack of motivation to get up some mornings, he is doing exceptionally well.

We had begun talking daily a couple of months ago, and him being back in my life gave me firmer footing to feel the peace that I now feel. He will soon be embarking on his own journey, and while I am going to help with that in a big way, he is strong enough and mature enough to do it on his own. We are very similar, and our bond is growing stronger every day.

Channing just graduated from the US Navy Basic Training in Great Lakes, IL. He signed on for five years with the Navy to be a Machinist Mate, and he has a solid plan for his future. He graduated high school this year, and while I wasn't there, I knew that he walked across that stage proud and able.

He, also, is an extremely strong young man, and a son I can truly say I am proud of. He will serve his country well, and will stand beside me, as I can with my own father, as a Veteran. And to be proud of being in that select company.

As I write this, he will be shipping out to Japan, to work onboard the U.S. Ronald Regan aircraft carrier. I worry about him, of course, but I couldn't be prouder. We talk at least once or twice a week, when our schedules line up, and we have bonded over shared experiences now, more than anything else.

Riley is still in high school and living with his mother and her husband in Texas. He is an exceptional athlete and does very well in school. He is the starting quarterback at his high school. But his real passion is art.

He is extremely gifted, just like his uncle Jasper, and his grandmother, my mother. He and I have not talked much in quite a while, but I hope he knows that I will always love him, and that even though I haven't been in his life like I always wanted, he has always been in my thoughts and prayers.

We began slowly talking again a couple of weeks ago, and while it's going slow, I'm being careful to not push him, or put too much on him. One day he will read this book, and hopefully understand why I did what I did. It's not an excuse, and I own what I've done, but it's an answer to him questioning if it was because of him. It was not.

All of my children are exceptional and perfect. My mistakes are mine alone and are the response to events I couldn't control. My job now, as their father, who has finally found peace and healing, is to repair those relationships, and take care of my responsibilities. I do that every day now.

The three little kids here in Maryland are well adjusted and thriving. I am trying my hardest to be back in their lives, as much as Priscilla will allow me. Our relationship is extremely rocky today, but I'm hoping as time goes by, it will get better.

It will get better because I am better. She still doesn't see who I am, or what I think and feel, but she does the best she knows how to do.

She is still extremely successful in her career and has spent the last 15 months taking care of the children by herself, with no support from me.

I'm working diligently to change that right now, but she has always been one to hold tenaciously to a grudge, and it will take a very long time to be cordial to each other. I hope one day we can be friends. I came to a realization not very long ago that has helped me to forgive Priscilla after I thought it was impossible to do so.

And that realization is that Priscilla does everything that she does, and to everyone that she pushes away, because she lives in a state of fear that even I don't comprehend.

252

I learned to sit back and look at her objectively, and I figured out that she is scared of almost everything. Failure, success, losing everyone, but keeping people close.

Allowing people in. Allowing the kids to have their own lives and minds.

She controls because she is so afraid of losing everything.

When I figured that out, it was a lot easier to forgive her. And ask for forgiveness in return. I know that she is almost incapable of forgiveness, but all I can do is forgive on my end, and try to remember why she does what she does, and why she is what she is.

When I accept her, it makes our interactions much easier.

So, recently, she and I finalized our divorce. She gave me joint custody of all three children, and I am working extremely hard to repair those relationships. We go to bi-monthly therapy sessions with the girls.

I hope, in the next six to nine months, to have a home and stability for them to spend half of their time. I hope one day that all of my children will be able to call my home-their home.

In the meantime, I am doing everything I can to assure everyone who I am responsible for has a brighter future. It's all I can do, and it's all that I am focused on.

Ruth Scott, I have found out recently has been married for a number of years and has three boys. I contacted her to ask her to read her part in this book, and she gave me positive feedback, which I expected completely. I can tell she hasn't changed a bit in the 22 years since I broke her heart. She is a shining light for God in a dark world. We no longer correspond beyond her reading the sections about her, but I wish and pray for her every success.

253

Sara has had a very rough time in her life since we parted ways. While it was ugly and painful for us to separate, we probably should not have been together in the first place. As an 18-year-old girl, I held too much influence over her, which I took advantage of.

That fact has affected her life the same way my childhood affected my own. It is not all my fault, but I am far from blameless for the decisions she has made as an adult. We recently started talking again.

While at first it was hate-filled and painful on her part, I have shown her the man that God has made me to be today. As the days went by, and we started talking more and more, and she drew strength from my own recovery, I think she has seen some light in her own life.

I am not sure what the future holds for Sara, but I know, with no hesitation, that she has the strength to overcome anything. She just needs to see that for herself.

She has amazing parents; whose lessons imparted to me during the short time we were together still resonate with me.

The other factor in this is our son. He is 13 years old now and doesn't have a strong father figure in his life. He doesn't know where he comes from. I hope that changes one day, but I will never push for it, or take it over from Sara.

I can only be here, steadfast, and for whatever she needs. Now that I know that our son is biologically mine, I will be here for the rest of my life for whatever he needs, when he needs it.

That's all I can do.

When he reads this, I hope he knows that while I didn't expound on his mom's and my time together, per her request, those months together changed me.

If it weren't for Sara, I would have not found God the way I did.

And God changing me in that jail cell, made me lose her.

But today, I am in such a better place, that the years in-between almost don't mean anything. It's hard to put words to.

But I am a much better man because of Sara, than not. I will always love her. But she has her own battles to overcome. I can only be strong for her, to be here for her, in whatever way I can. God will do the rest for her.

Cal Farley's Boy's Ranch is still doing what it has done for many years. It is changing young people's lives. I have been back out there a handful of times in the years since I drove away.

I recently took Riley and Channing there to see where their father grew up. It was an amazing visit, and all the smells and sights are exactly the same. God has touched that place and it will always be there. Anything I can do for the Ranch, I will do, happily. It will always be home.

Everyone else mentioned in this book is pretty much where I left them. My friends and family have come and gone without much wake in the sea of my life.

My father's family in Texas has had no contact with me in at least 14 years. I have no idea where they are or how they are doing. I cut off contact. Just as I did with my father's oldest four children. I know I have to pray to forgive them, but it will take time. I wish them all the best, but I have no interest in knowing any of them.

Everyone else, I just don't have any information on. Everyone in this book has made an impact on my life in one way or another, but one of the lessons I have recently learned is that I have to keep my circle very small. It's only for the best.

My best friend in life, Mary, is working herself to death in Texas. She is now the clinical director for all of the medically fragile foster kids in the state of Texas. She has finished raising three of her five children and is waiting for the last two to leave the house so that she can go on to do what she has always dreamed of doing.

I support her in everything that makes her happy, and I love her beyond belief. Many of us from the Ranch would do anything for her. She need only pick up a phone and she will have an army of brothers to do anything she needs. I'm pretty sure we could hide the bodies pretty well if that's what she needed.

She has read every word of this book as I've written it, and while nothing in it was a surprise to her, she nonetheless gave complete support.

Like my sister Venus, Mary is one of the strongest women I know, and I marvel at what she has been through. She is an inspiration for so many, whether she realizes it or not. We talk every single day, sometimes multiple times. She is another rock for me, and I am trying to be her strength as well.

Except for Jasper, I have known her longer than anyone else in my life. She saved me, and I hope that one day, I can do something similar for her.

My absolute best guy friend, Danny, who I haven't spoken of much in this book at his request is here with me every day.

We have spent the last few years together, working and laughing, talking, and bonding. He is an amazingly generous man, and one of my favorite people on this planet.

He is devoted to his children, and, even though he is younger than me, I look up to him as an amazing example of a man. He is my rock most days, as well as the rest of the circle. We all speak every day, and I'm blessed beyond belief to know them all.

Without the Circle, I would not be here today. And this story would not have been told.

The last word I got from Jane, just a few weeks ago, solidified my ability to move on from her. She is dating again and growing her business. The wounds I created in myself from pushing her away only strengthened me, not debilitated me, as they would have done even two months ago.

At times with Jane, I felt so strong and steady for her. And at others, I was afraid she would see through the façade and see what a real mess I was. Before I could be good for her, I had to be good for myself.

We had all the tools to be the most successful couple, a real power couple, but I wanted it too fast, and too hard. I pushed too much. I pushed past her reticence to make it healthy, and in doing so, I lost her.

Now, my only wish is for her happiness. I am setting my own life right, and getting the kids back is one part of that. A part I am working very hard on at the moment.

I also know, now, that Jane and I were not meant to be. She was as close to perfect as I have ever known, but looking back on our time together, we still weren't compatible in many ways.

Physically, we put so much pressure on it being perfect that it was far from it. Jane has her own demons as well. She was extremely healthy, but almost too much. Her boundaries were not boundaries, they were walls that she refused to tear down.

She told me once that she always ran away from anything that looked good for her life. That is something she is going to have to learn to overcome. I also know, at her age, that she still loves the night life, and in many ways was

257

sheltered and repressed for a long time. I am afraid that she may take the transitions in life very badly.

Any man with her at that time may get very hurt, whether she means to or not. So, it wasn't meant to be, and that's quite alright. I learned so very much from her. And I will be forever grateful for that. Because if it weren't for Jane, I wouldn't be the man I am today.

I also completely believe that my twin flame is out there. That there is a woman that God made just for me. I am not going to worry about her until God puts her in my life, and I'm not going to get back into another relationship until that time comes.

When you put your future and your life into God's hands, He gives you peace, instead of worry. I have that peace now. And I will let you know the real secret about God.

He knows us much better than we know ourselves.

As of this writing, I have spent the last several months alone, not wanting to be in a relationship.

But God knew my heart. I have not prayed for a special person this whole time. But God didn't need me to pray for what He wanted to give me.

When I closed out the previous chapter, I let some time go by before finishing up this manuscript. In that time, I have been alone, and getting stronger.

But six months ago, a simple salutation in the most innocent of ways and places set forth a quiet, barely perceptible chain of events that only God could orchestrate. The odds of this specific, and noticeably short introduction had God giving me what could be the greatest gift I have ever seen. I will not go into specifics, because even a breath of wind could cause this blessing to slip out of my hands.

But let me just say this. Everything I never knew I needed; God knew. He knew she would have to be an artist, a musician, a creative soul. She would have to love the Lord with all of her heart. She would have been through her own journey. And she would take my breath away with a smile.

God knew, and the odds meant nothing to Him. God made me say hello to a red-headed beauty six months ago, and ever so slowly, we have opened up to each other. My heart is full. And I never asked for it. And she didn't, either. This is a two-way miracle. And that's perfect as well.

And I am convinced more than anything that she will unconditionally love me for me, and allow me to be the intense, emotional person I am, but will partner with me through this life, and be worthy of the love I have learned though all of this to give, incessantly.

My gift for words, and her many gifts for art and music and just being an amazingly loving woman, will push us to what God wants for all of his children.

Our purposes to be fulfilled.

To use His gifts that He gives us to help each other. I'm still learning that lesson, and I know, that no matter how perfect someone seems, it's really up to me, to love myself enough to be secure for whoever God puts in my life.

I've messed this up too many times to keep letting it happen. Soon, I'm just going to shrug, tell God that He can use me as a bachelor just as easily as a married man. And leave it to Him to decide.

I also know I have to focus on myself and allow the time it takes for the healing to happen. I know that I can never lean on even the most perfect of women for my wholeness.

Another big thing has been happening in my life for the last couple of months.

I have learned that I am a really good man. That I am finally proud of the man that God created through this journey He started me on.

And that journey, and the experiences I gained have helped several friends in their own journey. I answer the phone six or seven times a day now for friends and acquaintances that need a good word. A gentle reminder to put their faith in God and see in themselves what He sees in them. They need someone who is following his own dream to give them hope to follow their own.

And God has put these people in my life now to do just that. To be, for the first time in my life, the support for others, rather than needing it myself.

The gift of that is beyond measure. And not for me. None of this is for me, or from me. I tell my friends every day that if I tried to tell them the right thing, I would fail.

I have done that, and I failed 100% of the time. Now, it is God's words, working through me, and allowing me to be the city on the hill. The beacon in the dark for several friends now, and who knows how many people who read these words later.

I am following my dreams, and I am doing it in the most beautiful place on the planet, Southern Maryland. Every road in this part of the country is like a picture on a postcard. I marvel daily why I ever left. Everything I love is right here.

I'm meeting new people and working diligently in therapy to hold onto this fragile peace and happiness I have found. But I know there is so much more in store. I can feel God pulling me to a new purpose. I don't know what that purpose is yet, but I feel it's coming soon. As I write this, God is moving in my life. Again, I don't know where I'm going, but I give it to God to get me there.

But the real miracle of this story is the day I decided to sit down and write it, the 5th of July 2019. I was in the deepest, darkest place in my life, but I knew in the middle of my broken soul, that by the time I finished it, it would have a happy ending.

And that happy ending is this: no matter what life throws at me from here on out, I will face it with the determination and strength I have earned through this life so far. I am completely happy to be alone right now because I know that I am not alone. I am a man of God, and I will no longer apologize for that. I have a real chance at being with my mirror soul. I know who I am now. I have gained wisdom and insight, as well as a solid willpower of my own. I am finally at peace.

I am finally a man I can be proud of.

God made this man. And I am a good man, finally. I am still a storyteller. But truth rules my life now. I no longer have to use lies as a defense mechanism for people to like me. Because now, I like me. I know with all of my heart now that God loves me, and that is more than enough.

I have come to see my life story for the good, rather than the bad. I realized that I have lived my life with a soundtrack playing that I couldn't always hear. The music of my life has been up and down, different genres, different tunes. But there has been a conductor, a DJ, who has made the music play. God has molded a life from these experiences that I can be proud of when I focus on the good, rather than react to the bad.

I am right where I am supposed to be, and future possibilities make me feel excitement and curiosity. I have joy, and I know what I am going to spend the rest of my life achieving.

The stories I have in my mind will find their way to paper, and hopefully to the hearts of everyone who has read this story and wants to see the glimpses of what comes next through my writing.

The truths I have learned will help those caught in the same hole I was in, and those whose lives have been harsh, and unyieldingly kicked them in the teeth, will see that you can get through it, as hard as that road is to walk.

They will realize that there was a time when they, too, sat on top of a brush and tree covered hill, gazing miles into the distance, at a road that symbolized the life they could only imagine, and even if it took half a lifetime, they will find themselves, one day, staring back and seeing what exactly has brought them from that day to this.

They will see that while we cannot do any of it alone, alone is what we have to learn to accept, to find our own happiness. That we can't rely on anyone else to find that for us. It sound contradictory, I know. We are all connected, yet we need to learn to be ok being alone. The one usually comes before the other, in a happy life.

It's not that you should want to be alone. It's that you should be happy either way.

That was very hard for me to figure out. I always felt that I had to have a partner. But the truth is, I'm not good at relationships. I'm hopefully getting a lot closer. But for now, at least, I'm better off figuring out my own path.

I cherish it now. I'm happy and have peace either way.

And that's where the miracle lies.

But there is one last thing for a peaceful life.

We are hardwired in our minds to need a belief in something bigger than ourselves, and a goal to strive towards. You have to absolutely follow your dreams. There is no other way.

I have learned to be grateful for all that I have, and all that I am. I could have ended my life a couple of times, but here I am, telling this story, and hoping that it helps someone else find their way to the peace and light I now possess.

Some will find who was made just for them, and many others will be content to be completely alone, surrounded by the many mistakes they had made in life, but everyone will have a chance to truly live.

Living, and loving; well, that's the other real miracle.

We are all connected in this world and what one feels, will be felt by many, in some way, without anyone realizing it. That connection, that energy, is what we should focus on, as there is no pain, no bad memories, and no horrible relationships in that energy. Call it what you want. Believe in whatever you want. But don't deny that we are all connected. I call it God. Others have called it a thousand things before. I'm sure, in the difficult times ahead for the planet, many more names for it will arise.

But now, I look around this coffee shop and I have a desire for everyone around me to feel what I feel at this moment. I can see all that connects us.

And in the stories in my mind, and the stories I see acted out all around me, the final truth is this: we must all learn to love.

It's in love that we find peace. It's in the relationships we are given in life where we are given the chance to act out that love, and in doing so, connect to the world in the only way that matters. With each other.

It's such a paradox, that we have to learn to be happy alone, but at the same time to see and have faith in the energy that connects us all. And to use that energy for good.

But the truth is, and here is the secret of this story, dear readers:

When you can achieve both, a singular miracle happens.

You learn your purpose.

And you find real joy.

I'm going to finish this now, put my things away, and leave this coffee shop knowing the peace and joy I have now came from a place of hurt and pain, extreme abuse, and neglect.

And when I found freedom from it, I learned I could do anything.

I will change the world.

And I hope these words, in some small way, changes your world.

I drive away from this story now, hearing the tires crunch on the blacktop of the road under me. I feel the invisible lines of love connecting all of us, from my heart to all others.

Two teardrops fall from my eyes and I press the gas pedal, driving forward into the future.

The story is now yours.

For me, I will never look back.

J. L. Fox

Lexington Park, MD

July 5-October 5, 2019

Please stay tuned for my next book, "Had I Not Chosen." It is available now, from Watertower Hill Publishing. I hope that it will show each of you the beauty and wonder that God gives us in our relationships, whether we choose them or not. Whether we choose life, or not. Whether we choose to save the world, or not.

Until then, God bless each of you who embarked on this journey with me. There is so much more to come.

Resources:

www.jlfoxbooks.com

www.watertowerhillpublishing.com

www.beautyafterbruises.org

https://cptsdfoundation.org/

https://www.reddit.com/r/CPTSD/

https://www.outofthestorm.website/

https://www.youtube.com/watch?v=95ovIJ3dsNk

https://www.developingchild.harvard.edu/take-the-ace-quiz

"The Body Keeps the Score: Brain, Mind, and Body in the Healing of Trauma" by Bessel van der Kolk M.D.

"PSYCHIATRIC HOSPITALS TRAINED IN TRAUMA AND DISSOCIATION" **

- **Sheppard Pratt Health System**: *The Trauma Disorders Program* | Towson, MD

- **River Oaks Hospital**: *Trauma Disorders* | New Orleans, LA

- **McLean Hospital:** *Dissociative Disorders and Trauma Program* | Belmont, MA

- **Psychiatric Institute of Washington (PIW)**: *The Center* | Washington D.C., MD*

- **Forest View Hospital:** Trauma Program | Grand Rapids, MI (unsure of current status of their individual inpatient unit for Trauma Disorders; trauma care may be co-habitant with other patients; does have specialized PHP) *

- **Del Amo:** *The Trauma Recovery Program* | Torrance, CA* (cites following the Colin Ross Trauma Model)

- **UBH Denton:** *The Ross Institute for Trauma* | Denton, TX (formerly the program at Timberlawn, nurses and staff made the transfer as well; is a Colin A Ross Institute Trauma Program using his Trauma Model) *

- **The Trauma Center at JRI:** Brookline, MA* (only offers residential treatment to adolescents aged 12-22, but also offers and abundance of other therapeutic opportunities particularly after evaluation; follows research of Bessel van der Kolk. Recent conversations suggest that, because of an overly complex assessment process, unless you live locally, this may not be a viable option.)

- **Two Rivers Behavioral Health System** | Kansas City, MO (no longer has specialized, inpatient trauma treatment; no longer sure about PHP/IOP programs either) *

*Several of these facilities have partial (PHP) and/or intensive out-patient programs as well.

This is only the current list of **inpatient facilities. There *are* some other locations that offer residential care, acute stabilization (3-5 days), or solely PHP/IOP. If you are interested in knowing those options, please contact any of the websites above for that list. These programs are constantly changing and tend to be more unstructured, smaller in size, and more expensive and unregulated (residential programs specifically), but if you are in need of *some* kind of treatment and none of these are available to you, any of the resources above will happily help you see if any others like this are viable."

(Taken from www.beautyafterbruises.org, 2019)

Epilogue

When I finished the story that this book tells, I wanted to wait a year, and then publish it. And in that year, I wanted to let the miracles and lessons that God has given me to shape my life, and see what I would see.

I want to give this one last update, one year later, to prove that it wasn't all for naught.

That the man that God made through the story told here, was still the same man on the day that I finished it.

So, that's what I am doing here. At some point, I need to just finish this, and you, constant reader, can see where I am, like every other author.

So, 12 months later, it's now the beginning of October, 2020.

Every day of the last year, I have woken up early, before work starts, and wrote. I finished my first fictional novel. And I am, as of today, ¾ finished with the second. That's almost 3 novels in 18 months. Not too bad for a short, fat kid.

I have spent the entirety of the last year getting stronger. Stronger than I have ever been, both physically and mentally. I have pushed myself every single day to do the things that most other people won't do, or can't do.

I have gotten physically more fit by walking more than six or eight miles a day, working out at the gym three or four times a week, and being so proud of the strides I have made to take care of myself in every way possible.

I have continued in my therapy, and now, when I see my therapist, it's just to make sure that I am making the decisions I make daily from a place of health, and not reactions to negative emotions.

That, more than anything, had helped me get stronger.

And so, yes, one year later, I am still so proud of myself.

I am also somewhere I never expected to be living. As the relationship I mentioned at the end of the story blossomed, I realized that she lived very close to my mother's family in New England. Over several months earlier this year, we got to know each other, and visited each other infrequently. I was working on getting the little kids at my home more often, and writing, as well as working my day job.

We took it slow, got to know each other deeply, and prayed together about it. She was going through her own journey, and I encouraged her in that. After several months, we decided that I would move up to New England, if a job worked out, my family agreed, and God made it happen. All 3 stipulations worked out, and in July of this year, I headed north.

One thing that I mentioned in this story, is my time visiting my mother's family here. I love them all deeply, and feel a real connection to the area. As the months of July and August came and went, I got to know the area even better. I absolutely love it here. It's even more beautiful than Southern Maryland, if that's possible.

I got to know Red's parents and friends and family very well. There were many hurdles to overcome, but we tried our best to do them together, and try to build something. I shared all of my dreams, goals, and the journey I had traveled. She reciprocated, and shared the same.

I didn't know, at that time, that just because those dreams had not come to fruition yet, she saw them as lies. And that happens a lot. And it's one of the best weapons that the enemy has over us, right before the biggest breakthroughs. She, unwittingly, became a tool of the enemy against me.

You see, she wasn't as far on her journey as I was. I think that if she had taken a year to be alone, she would have figured out what she wanted in life, and things would have worked out differently. And she would have found the wisdom that I was given when I took the time and energy to find it.

But that didn't happen. And that's ok. At the end, she figured some of it out, as did I, and we parted ways. It wasn't as traumatic as other times, and it wasn't sad or depressing. At least not for me. I can't answer that for her. She saw everything I did with her as abuse and lies.

And what she did over the next several months, showed me very clearly that she was not the person she made herself out to be, and the fact that she can't see the real truth of things, I can't really do anything about. I refuse to control people like that, or at least attempt to, anymore.

It wastes my time, and theirs.

She launched a campaign against me, trying to show those I love in my life, that I was a horrible person. She dug more into my past, and talked to the women mentioned in this book, who had their own problems with me, because we all know that people need to feel justified in their mindsets. It makes them feel better, and that they are seeing truth. The pirate reached out to her after our breakup, and I'm sure they had several lovely conversations about how evil I am.

What they don't know, is that two or three people seeing evil in a person, evil does not make.

People tend to need a bad guy in their story, so that it justifies the bad things they, themselves, do.

Her age, lack of experience, and general low self-esteem showed that she wasn't ready for a relationship with someone like me. And that's ok.

She is still an amazing person, with gifts that most people would die for. What she does with her life, is none of my business. I only wish her the best, and I want to tell her thank you, right here.

I think, that what she didn't realize, is that this book points out the things she believes much more clearly than anything she could ever do or say against me. Or what anyone else can say, frankly.

I WAS a horrible person. I lied to everyone, and used people. I did it out of being in survival mode for so many years. It wasn't until the end of this story that I started to live a different way, and see myself as a different man.

All she can do now is prove the point of the miracle of what God did for me, and to me.

And in that, we have such a powerful example, given by circumstances, that God, Himself, gets the glory in all of this. And whatever comes from it.

So, after a night, and only a single night, of seeing how she saw me, I realized some real truths, once again.

I am STILL strong, independent, and have been made into a really good man. I have only deepened my relationship with God, my family, and my Circle.

I still have the peace He gave me over the last couple of years. I am still whole, happy, and have purpose and joy every day. He did add one more thing to me, though.

He gave me an understanding of why people, including myself, have done, and continue to do, the things they do. It helps me to find forgiveness, and I see intentions and emotions earlier than I ever have before.

For instance, at least a month before Red and I split up, I saw it all coming. I started to set boundaries around my heart, so that I wouldn't be hurt when what I knew was going to happen, finally happened. And that understanding, I call it wisdom.

I thank God every day for that wisdom.

So, that was that. I have a home that I have worked very hard to have. I have filled it with things that are completely me, and the kids all have room here. But it's not my final destination.

My goals and dreams are still as lofty as I can make them. I continue to study, learn, write, and consume everything I can for the peace that God has gifted me with. It makes every day a blessed day.

But God knew that sometimes I feel lonely. So, He made two other connections for me over the last year that have added more than I can ever thank Him for. He gave me an old friend back, and a new love here with me today.

When I was at Boys Ranch, decades ago, I knew a girl named Alexis. She was there with her brother, and both of them were bright spots. While I didn't know her as well as I knew her brother, she was still an acquaintance. She played sports very well, and we would talk about that, more than anything else. Again, we weren't close, weren't in the same groups, and I was three years older.

But as I moved back to Maryland last year, we re-connected. She is hugely successful, has a wonderful family, and her husband does things in the military that I am oh, too familiar with.

Over the same last 12 months, she and I have become as close as I am to Mary. We speak every day, and we cross-connect both of our careers, and our goals and dreams. She gets the deep depths of life like I do. She is certainly not a surface swimmer. We have talked for hours about intentions, and positive mindsets. I'm not sure how or what to call what she is now, but she is amazingly successful in the world of Sports Science, and Sports Psychology. She has connections all the way up into the Olympic world, as well as colleges and universities all over the country. She has her own business, her own e-learning school online, and works harder than anyone else I know. But she is also amazingly open with me, and I am with her as well.

She is a beautiful guide, but also needs advice here and there. Our relationship is very back and forth, but it's strong, and will be there the rest of our lives. I love her as a great friend, and look forward to watching her family grow.

I am still very close with the entire Circle as well. We all speak every day. My two oldest sons are now a part of that Circle, and everyone else is doing well.

Mary and I still speak every single day, and her and her family are coming to New England to visit me for Thanksgiving. I am very excited to see all of them.

The second thing that God blessed me with is a new love of my life.

Her name is Clover, and she is a trained comfort/therapy dog from a group here in New England called HeroPups.

They approved me to have her, and she has brought joy to my life that I wasn't expecting. She is amazingly smart, loyal, and funny. She is a golden retriever, and except for leaving hair all over everything, she is my new constant companion.

We walk several times a day here in beautiful New England, and we were made for each other. We recently drove down to Maryland to see the little kids, and she was just perfect in the car, the entire way. She also likes to listen to True Crime Podcasts in the car.

She told me so herself.

And that's where I stand. I am happy being alone again, or at least alone with a whole circle of amazing people I speak to daily, and a beautiful puppy dog always by my side.

And, as I've come to know God, I know that He will put real love in my life in ways that I can't even imagine. I just sit here, patiently awaiting His continued blessings, and when He chooses her, He will put her in my life. Until then, I press forward.

I am ok, no matter what.

Because now I have peace, passion, and purpose. I am always writing, communicating, and making my dreams and goals reality.

And that's all that I can hope for. To have amazing days, every single day. I pray and hope that these days continue for the rest of my life, and that I can always give back, however I can.

That's my biggest dream and goal.

To be able to give back.

Whatever that looks like, and however God leads me to do it. I am His. And I am full of joy to do it.

I pray for you all, wish you the greatest joy, and want nothing but good things for this world. I am working every day to make this a better world, however I can.

I owe it to everything I've been given back, to return it to the world, in any way that I can.

Because it was first given to me.

J.L Fox

October, 2020

Made in the USA
Middletown, DE
14 April 2023